Songwriting

Songwriting

Methods, Techniques and Clinical Applications for
Music Therapy Clinicians, Educators and Students

Edited by Felicity Baker and Tony Wigram

Jessica Kingsley Publishers
London and Philadelphia

Ethical guideline

The therapeutic methods and techniques defined and described in this book are for use by qualified clinical music therapy practitioners and students in training who have completed or are undertaking recognized clinical training.

First published in 2005
by Jessica Kingsley Publishers
116 Pentonville Road
London N1 9JB, UK
and
400 Market Street, Suite 400
Philadelphia, PA 19106, USA

www.jkp.com

Library of Congress Cataloging in Publication Data

Songwriting : methods, techniques and clinical applications for music therapy clinicians, educators, and students / edited by Felicity Baker and Tony Wigram.
    p. cm.
Includes bibliographical references and index.
ISBN-13: 978-1-84310-356-1 (pbk.)
ISBN-10: 1-84310-356-7 (pbk.)
1. Music therapy--Case studies. I. Baker, Felicity, 1970- II. Wigram, Tony.
ML3920.S726 2005
615.8'5154--dc22

2005001861

British Library Cataloguing in Publication Data

A CIP catalogue record for this book is available from the British Library

ISBN 978 1 84310 356 1

Printed and bound in the United States by
Thomson-Shore, Inc.

Contents

List of Tables

List of Figures

FOREWORD

Soundtracks of our life

Even Ruud

Music therapists have always recognized songs and singing as one of their main approaches within their work. Along with improvisation, listening, composing and performing, songs have had their natural place in the music therapist's tool-box as a way of expressing and performing aspects of oneself as part of a process towards better health. But what about songwriting? Can we say that the actual making of the song by the client or the process of co-creating a song together with the therapist has gained full recognition among the repertoire of methods in music therapy?

I can only answer for myself that after reading this book on songwriting, I must declare my own ignorance of what seems to stand out as one of the most powerful methods in music therapy. In hindsight, at the time when I was active as a music therapist, I had not fully recognized my own attempts at songwriting as songwriting, and instead labelled it 'free improvisation' or 'musical plays'. Regardless of whatever theoretical or clinical tradition you work in, this book will enable you to see new possibilities in many music therapy situations. As a method, songwriting transcends the many theoretical traditions that feed the work of music therapists. Both cognitive and psychodynamic discourses can operate well within this medium, just as environmental and resource-oriented perspectives inform and expand the possibilities of actions afforded by the production of songs.

From childhood on, we all relate to songs and songwriting in a personal way. Children improvise with their voices, create mock-versions of familiar songs, and engage in a host of changing forms of identifications with songs and singers on their way to adulthood. The song text often provides an early experience of how to symbolically represent the world, and of how we can use metaphors to understand the meaning of what is happening to us.

Singer-songwriters are the heroes of today's popular culture. Songs are chronicles, not only of the private and personal, but also of everyday occurrences and political issues. The current plurality of genres and styles of songwriting have made this musical cultural form into an ever-present soundtrack of our lives. The art songs, folk songs, religious songs, popular songs and songwriting have long historical traditions. There is a song for everyone and for everything.

This familiarity, our intimate knowledge of this cultural form, gives songs and songwriting a special place among the methods of music therapy. Throughout this book, we meet numerous examples of how music therapists have become masters of appropriating popular culture in order to help clients formulate, ventilate, express and communicate some of their deepest wishes and thoughts. It seems like the song gives the client a new context, a freedom and strength to bypass his or her own vulnerability. The song form not only *affords* a range of possibilities for self-expression, but it equally *allows* one to touch on and warm to themes and relationships which have been deeply-frozen for a long time. Songwriting provides an aesthetic context inviting clients to explore, within a new play-frame, their own life, their possibilities, their losses and their aspirations.

INTRODUCTION

Songwriting as Therapy

Tony Wigram and Felicity Baker

Songs have long been part of a music therapist's tool kit. When used in therapy sessions across the lifespan they can provide safety, support, stimulation or sedation. They can assist people to reflect on their past, present or future, to make contact with unconscious thought processes, to confront difficulties within their intrapersonal experiences and their interpersonal relationships, and to project their feelings into music. Songs can also be used in facilitating the development or redevelopment of functional skills including physical, cognitive or communication functions. Within groups, songs assist in developing group cohesiveness, encouraging social interaction and providing group support. Further, songs can facilitate the development of the therapeutic relationship between client and therapist. Importantly, songs can provide opportunities for clients to experience joy during times when they might find joyous occasions few and far between. As Bruscia so aptly states:

> Songs are ways that human beings explore emotions. They express who we are and how we feel, they bring us closer to others, they keep us company when we are alone. They articulate our beliefs and values. As the years pass, songs bear witness to our lives. They allow us to relive the past, examine the present, and to voice our dreams of the future. Songs weave tales of our joys and sorrows, they reveal our innermost secrets, and they express our hopes and disappointments, our fears and triumphs. They are our musical diaries, our life-stories. They are the sounds of our personal development. (Bruscia 1998, p.9)

The role and value of songs

If songs can hold an important place in therapy, and songwriting is an effective media in therapy, which is the primary theme of this book, then where do songs stand as a musical style and cultural phenomena through the historical development of humankind? Perhaps the easiest starting point here is that 'Music began with singing' (Sachs 1969, p.4). Back in the ancient times, the two main purposes of singing – both of which are actually very relevant to music therapy and to songwriting – were defined as logogenic – where the style was a monotonous 'sing-song' giving a primary focus of attention on the words – or pathogenic – where the style was less concerned with the words of a song, but rather with discharging tension, force, irritation, and was defined as passion-born. During these ancient times, songs were primarily a vehicle for story-telling, and the heroes of the Greeks in the periods ninth to seventh centuries BC sang songs, usually at weddings and funerals, accompanied by the lyre (Lang 1941, p.6). During early history and the middle ages, song singing was primarily related to religious worship, and certainly intended to chant the liturgy in a less emotional and pure way. Songs were not supposed to be the containers of emotions, or stories, other than those connected with religious rites.

It was during and at the end of the medieval era that drama began to take a place in religious worship, and medieval lyric poetry developed by the troubadours in France saw new developments in the role of song. Wandering poets and singers carried news and fascinating stories, and secular music saw the development of opera – at first rejected as a 'satanic' activity by the conservatives in the church, where the style and function of music in worship was carefully defined and controlled. Of course the troubadours were stepping into a very new realm of music – romantic song with the theme of love, and worship of love. How little has changed over the centuries since the heyday of the troubadours in the period 1150–1210; throughout the renaissance, classical, romantic and twentieth-century periods, songs have become increasingly important for the precise functions for which they were originally developed – telling stories, reflecting emotions and enhancing worship.

This introduction would become too lengthy to start a detailed exploration of the relevance of song to the development of both music and humankind, and there is a complex history of development involved, from madrigals to song cycles, ballads to rap. Popular song continues to capture the hearts and minds of every generation, as well as acting as a mirror in reflecting the cultural, political and philosophical attitudes at the time. We use them for love and anger, in peace and war, in despair and in hope, to celebrate and to protest. Perhaps the important issue here is to offer a definition of song, of songwriting and then of songwriting in music therapy.

Stainer and Barrett (1875) in their *Dictionary of Musical Terms* described song as 'A piece of music for voice or voices, whether accompanied or unaccompanied, or the act or art of singing'. Their definition presents a simple and clear perspective and relates to song both as an object, and as a form of musical expression. Songwriting is not really defined in dictionaries, except the reference to songsters and songwriter in *The New Groves Dictionary of Music and Musicians* (Sadie 1980, p.524). Here, a songster is identified as a 'black American musician of the post-reconstruction era who performed a wide variety of ballads, dance-tunes, reels and minstrel songs...to his own banjo or guitar accompaniment' (p.721). Songwriter is specified as a 'composer (or lyricist) who writes songs' (p.722). The songwriter emerged in the 1920s and 1930s as a musician who could earn their living solely from writing songs.

As the popularity of songs increased with the advent of record players, there was seen the emergence of a 'hit' which signified substantial sales. There also emerged a particular style of songwriting, sometimes by a single person, and sometimes by teams such as that of Rodgers and Hammerstein. This was simply a development of the old relationship between poet and musician, lyricist or librettist and composer, which has seen many famous partnerships. But the period when the songwriter style developed into singer-songwriter in the 1960s is significant for the role of songwriting in music therapy. Here there was a more clear evidence of the investment and ownership of the song, both in its creation, and the idiosyncratic way the songwriter performs it. These days, non-performing songwriters remain largely unknown and unacknowledged, whereas the performers stamp both the song, and their 'interpretation' of it, with their identity. In therapy, the identity of the person, in the song, is what captures the essence of the technique – which is why it is interesting to see in the ensuing chapters how much emphasis on the part of the therapist is placed on the importance of the clients creating the song as much as possible from their own ideas, material and musical preference.

Songwriting as a method in therapy

Emerging from the use of songs within therapeutic contexts is the technique of songwriting. For many years, clinicians have been writing songs *for* clients and *with* clients to address various therapeutic goals. A distinction between these two broadly termed techniques is necessary as this book focuses primarily on the latter technique – writing songs *with* clients. Writing songs *for* clients refers to the clinician's composition of songs for a specific client, group of clients, or specific therapeutic purpose – whether this is for clients' psychological, emotional, social, physical, spiritual or communication needs. Through their university training, music therapy clinicians have highly developed abilities to compose songs that are stylistically age-appropriate and engaging for the specific client population, and are appropriately constructed to address the specific therapeutic needs of their clients.

In contrast, writing songs *with* clients serves a different purpose and is akin to the concept of music *as* therapy. Here, the process and product of writing a song within therapy sessions *is* the therapeutic intervention. The therapeutic effect is brought about through the client's creation, performance and/or recording of his or her own song. The therapist's role within the music therapeutic relationship is to facilitate this process ensuring that the client creates a composition that can be felt as owned by the client and expressive of his or her personal needs, feelings and thoughts.

Songs created within therapeutic contexts can be viewed in terms of process and product. They are evidence of the beginning, middle or end of a therapeutic process, or an entire therapeutic process in and of itself. Clients create songs that reflect feelings and thoughts felt or experienced at points during their treatment and are therefore documents of their therapeutic journey. Nevertheless, these creations are also artefacts, products that clients can revisit, share with others, and be evidence of mastery, creativity and self-expression.

The music therapy literature is abundant with case examples of the use of songwriting as therapy and there are a handful of research articles describing the method and outcomes of this approach to treatment. Other research has focused more on the experiences of clients who have used songwriting within their treatment. The documentation of the value of songwriting with children and adolescents who have cancer, blood disorders or undergoing bone marrow transplants is considerable, particularly in recent years (Abad 2003; Hadley 1996; Kennelly 1999; Ledger 2001; Robb 1996; Robb and Ebberts 2003a, 2003b; Slivka and Magill 1986; Turry 1999). By employing a variety of songwriting interventions, children and adolescents experiencing life-threatening illness have had opportunities to experience mastery (Abad 2003; Robb and Ebberts 2003a) and increase their self-esteem through their participation in positive hospital experiences (Hadley 1996; Kennelly 1999; Ledger 2001). In some cases, clinicians and researchers have observed reductions in these patients' anxiety, anger and tension (Robb and Ebberts 2003a; Slivka and Magill 1986; Turry 1999) and observed improvements in coping (Robb and Ebberts 2003a) and social interaction with others (Abad 2003; Robb 1996; Slivka and Magill 1986).

Similar therapeutic goals have been addressed through songwriting with adolescents who present with emotional difficulties. In particular, the expression of

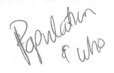

thoughts and feelings and enhanced self-esteem were rather common (Edgerton 1990; Goldstein 1990; Lindberg 1995; Robarts 2003). Robarts (2003) presents an interesting case of a girl who had been the survivor of sexual abuse and found that improvised songs were beneficial in allowing her client to express unconscious aspects of herself, acknowledge sadness and loneliness and develop confidence.

Edwards (1998) found that songwriting facilitated a change in perception of the hospital experience for children with burns whereas Fischer (1991) and Gfeller (1987) used songwriting for more functional outcomes – in order to learn concepts and for reading and writing skill development.

In the adult population, songwriting has also been implemented to address a range of needs for patients being treated for cancer or palliative care (O'Callaghan 1990, 1996), for patients with mental health issues (Ficken 1976; Montello 2003), for patients with traumatic brain injury (Glassman 1991), substance abuse patients (Freed 1987), and people in aged care facilities (Silber and Hes 1995). Again, the rationale for using songwriting approaches include the expression of thoughts and feelings (Glassman 1991; O'Callaghan 1990, 1996), developing insight and problem-solving skills (Glassman 1991; Montello 2003), providing emotional, spiritual and psychosocial support (Freed 1987; O'Callaghan 1990, 1996), and social interaction (Ficken 1976; Silber and Hes 1995).

Several structured and unstructured songwriting techniques were described in the literature. 'Fill-in-the-blank' techniques were frequently cited whereby key-words within a pre-composed song are 'blanked-out' and clients replace these with their own words (Freed 1987; Glassman 1991; Goldstein 1990; Robb 1996). A slightly modified version of fill-in-the-blank was also employed whereby additional verses to popular songs were created by the clients (Ficken 1976). By far the most frequently described intervention was that of song parody (Abad 2003; Edwards 1998; Ficken 1976; Freed 1987; Glassman 1991; Ledger 2001). In these cases, the original lyrics of a popular song chosen by the clients were replaced with their own lyrics while maintaining the melodic and harmonic frame and the genre of the song. These techniques seemed to be employed when clients needed a structured approach to facilitate the song creation. Schmidt (1983) argues that the song-form of the 12-bar blues song is also a useful frame for clients to write lyrics to as it creates a strong and definable structure.

Freely composed songs allow for more creativity and have been adopted as one approach for clients across broad age ranges and pathologies (Cordobés 1997; Edwards 1998; Gfeller 1987; Hadley 1996; Lindberg 1995; O'Callaghan 1990, 1996; Robb and Ebberts 2003a). Lindberg (1995) outlines one approach whereby a list of words is generated through free association and the client then identifies keywords. These keywords are then used for building lyrics to a song. Cordobés

(1997) provides a starting point for her clients by offering the topic of a specific emotion in which they then use to create lyrics for a song. Similarly, Gfeller (1987) gives her clients a theme to write about. Robb and Ebberts (2003a) incorporated the use of digital video recording, photos and artwork into the songwriting process to enhance its effect.

In employing a more psychoanalytically informed approach, improvised song creations were also present within the literature and generally focused on developing insight and expressing unconscious aspects of the self (Montello 2003; Robarts 2003), expressing uncomfortable emotions (Robarts 2003; Turry 1999), and developing confidence and a new sense of self (Robarts 2003).

While songwriting was generally reported as an intervention used in one-to-one therapy, a few authors have described its application within groups (Cordobés 1997; Edgerton 1990; Freed 1987; Robb 1996; Silber and Hes 1995) stating that the group experiences encourage social interaction, group cohesion and feelings of group supportiveness.

The focus of this book is to present a variety of applications of songwriting as therapy, with different clinical and non-clinical populations, with close attention to the method by which the intervention was undertaken. In preparation for the variety of methods, techniques and applications of songwriting in therapy, a provisional definition can be presented here of songwriting in music therapy as:

> The process of creating, notating and/or recording lyrics and music by the client or clients and therapist within a therapeutic relationship to address psychosocial, emotional, cognitive and communication needs of the client.

It is also important at this stage to clarify what is meant by 'method' and what is meant by 'technique'. Therapeutic methods are the approaches chosen by the therapist to achieve therapeutic change, and can be understood as the 'method' of work. Conversely, techniques are the 'tools and strategies', musical 'activities' and concrete therapist-initiated musical experiences which are integral to the success of the applied method. The vast majority of literature in music therapy has tended to focus on the therapeutic value and/or outcome of different forms of music therapy intervention with a variety of populations. It rarely explains (even in the broadest of terms) the method by which the intervention was undertaken, let alone procedural details or the techniques that were applied. The same conclusions can be drawn from the literature on songwriting cited above. There can be some explanations for this, with some issues being broadly methodological:

1. improvisational approaches, methods and techniques are spontaneous, and typically unsystematic

2. there is no consistency in the way methods are applied

3. clients' needs demand flexibility in any procedure

4. music therapy methods, even within taught models, vary widely.

Other issues, however, are of more philosophical or individual thinking:

1. we should not manualize our working method

2. some music therapists can't define their specific methods, because they were never really taught them, or have not tried to explain them

3. some music therapists regard their method as individual and unique, 'owned' by them, and therefore not replicable by others.

This may sound rather a hard critique on the profession, where some models of work are pretty well described, and certainly underpinned by strong theoretical foundations. In fact, the theoretical framework for music therapy is clearly an area of strength, and is well documented (Bruscia 1987, 1998; Davis, Gfeller and Thaut 1999; Priestley 1998; Ruud 1998; Stige 2002; Wigram, Pedersen and Bonde 2002). Therefore the issues raised above that might explain a lack of apparent evidence of detailed method reflect only the difficulty that may always have been present for both academics and clinicians to define clearly their method of work. Our contention is that this need not be so, and the ambition of this text is to contribute to the literature with a methods book that is grounded in clinical experience. As has so often happened in the past, theory has emerged from empirical experiences, and in this case methods and techniques will be defined and, it is hoped, formalized from empirical practice. Why should this be an important and relevant contribution at this stage in the development of music therapy? There are a number of reasons that relate to the education of music therapists, evidence-based practice and clinical governance, and future research in the field.

Students' requirements: music therapy education

Both trainers of music therapists and the students themselves increasingly expect to be able to teach or learn 'tried and tested' methods that they will place in their clinical repertoire. There is a paucity of therapy techniques in certain areas, and sometimes a lack of certainty in teaching. A model or approach often appears to reflect a 'trial and error' philosophy, notwithstanding that there are some broad principles in intervention to which all can subscribe. Students are often advised, or even encouraged to think, that they will develop their own 'method' and that there is no single or identifiable procedure for music therapy intervention which they can (or should) incorporate. This lack of specified technique is an inherent weakness, and shows up most in music therapy education where students may have expected to be taught valid and reliable techniques of intervention. Instead, they are left with a framework for therapeutic decision-making which is much more loosely connected to technique and method than they may have expected or deserve. This does not infer that we should be developing guaranteed but rigid procedures, or prioritized and exclusive intervention techniques. Not at all! As this book will demonstrate, there are several different ways to reach a goal, some quite similar, and others different. The teachers and students in music therapy are, nevertheless, entitled to expect greater clarity in therapeutic method and technique as the history develops.

Clinicians' requirements: evidence-based practice and clinical governance

From the perspective of the clinician, there is an increasing demand for therapists to describe and define the 'pill', or contents thereof that has such wondrous effects! In less poetic terms, we need to explain better what exactly it was we did that worked, and its purpose, based on clinical evidence, to explain why we should continue with an intervention modality. The requirements of evidence-based practice (EBP), and the way that they are implemented through clinical governance (CG), expect clinicians to apply therapeutic interventions which are supported by patient-reported, clinician-observed and research-based evidence. So the remarkable process and results of music therapy need to be presented in a detailed and understandable form not only to music therapy clinicians, music therapy educators and students in training, but also to members of other disciplines and purchasers of healthcare and educational services. This book follows on from *Improvisation* (Wigram 2004) where just such an attempt was made to describe specifically the techniques and methods that we use – both for teaching purposes and for the analysis and explanation of clinical process and outcome.

Researchers' challenges: future research into method

The demands of EBP and CG particularly relate to the presence or absence of evidence that an intervention is effective, valid and reliable. This book will not address these aspects of process and outcome research – it is not our intention to do that. But it is easier for future researchers to have a more clear starting point in addressing those aspects if there are clearly defined methods (supported by some anecdotal clinical examples) from which future studies can derive clinical outcomes. It is noticeable in other disciplines that studies, and particularly those concerned with evaluating or standardizing assessment and evaluation procedures, are beginning with a clearly defined method or procedure as a basis for the design.

At this stage in the development of the profession, it would be ambitious to expect that there would be an already defined and agreed procedure for applying songwriting as a method in music therapy. There has, to our knowledge, been no 'working group' or multi-centre research study intending to define and describe a common, generic procedure for songwriting, and it would be detrimental to attempt to impose one anyway. However, the chapters in this book are going to present a variety of styles that have emerged in an idiosyncratic way from different clinical populations and certainly within different cultures ranging through the US, Australia and Europe. What we will search for will be the similarities in style, method and technique as well as the unique differences. To that end, we presented our contributors with certain challenges.

Each chapter will offer an overview of the purpose/value/role of songwriting as a music therapy method and intervention with a specific population, referring where possible to its relevance for the therapeutic process and goals which could include:

- communication development/redevelopment
- self-expression or self-exploration
- life review
- coping and/or adjusting (for example, externalizing painful issues)
- developing/redeveloping cognitive abilities
- other therapeutic goals.

The methodological orientation of each contributor will be summarized, with attention to their therapeutic framework, addressing:

- the theoretical, psychological or health approaches by which interventions are influenced
- the rationale behind group or individual approaches to songwriting.

The main emphasis of each contribution will be directed towards describing in as much detail as possible the method and techniques used in the contributor's songwriting intervention including:

- how clients are introduced to the technique (is it during the first session, after development of rapport, at a certain stage within the therapy programme etc.)

- whether lyrics or music are created first

- how lyrics are created

- the method by which the music is written

- defining the length of the process and whether it occurs in a single session or over many sessions

- the genre of music/accompaniment style, and what patients seem to choose

- the development of a performance of the song

- the development of the song as a 'final product' and what happens to it

- techniques used in group songwriting

- aspects of a songwriting method that are important for clinicians when working with a specific population

- any criteria for the method to be indicated for a specific population

- any contraindications to consider when applying the method with a specific population.

Finally, in each chapter, contributors have presented an example or examples from their clinical practice to illustrate the method, the process and the outcome. Wherever possible, examples of song/lyric/melodic/harmonic material are included to make explicit the techniques utilized in clinical work, and there are notated songs in the book, with music and lyrics.

Introduction to the chapters

Amelia Oldfield has years of experience in child assessment and child development centres working with children with autistic spectrum disorders, Asperger's Syndrome and other pervasive developmental disorders. In Chapter 1, Oldfield and Christine Franke (psychotherapist and co-author) describe the more spontaneous process of improvised song creation and how it can be applied to assess the emotional world of a child within a psychiatric assessment unit. Oldfield and Franke clearly describe the way the music therapist introduces the technique and what the music therapist does to facilitate the song creation. They present techniques that musically 'heighten' the effect of the improvised song, and various musical and verbal techniques to deal with the non-responsive, the avoidant, the aggressive or the rigid child. These two experienced clinicians offer important explanations as to how children's improvised song creations reveal the psychological and emotional state of the children seen within a Kleinian frame.

Alongside Oldfield, Emma Davies also works in child and adolescent mental health services, and the focus of her chapter is on her work with emotionally and behaviourally disturbed children and adolescents. In describing her method of work, Davies, in keeping with the theoretical ideas of Winnicott, emphasizes the need for creating and developing the right environment prior to introducing the songwriting method. Another interesting aspect of Davies' work is her inclusion of listening to popular music within the music therapy sessions to trigger ideas for the creation of the music. The concept of 'word painting' as a technique to stimulate the creation of lyrics is carefully described by Davies and is a useful technique which could be applied with other populations.

Philippa Derrington describes the application of songs, song improvisation and song composition when working with teenagers with emotional and behavioural difficulties in a mainstream school in England. This field of work is not where one typically encounters music therapy, but songwriting has a strong attraction and motivation for teenagers who live with the pop culture. Her chapter examines the role and application of songwriting with students in order to address needs such as: reductions in tension, anxiety and challenging behaviour; the development of positive self-image and independence; the development of insight; and an increased awareness of the self and others.

Toni Day's clinical interests and expertise is in working with women who have been abused as children. In a collaborative project with a social worker, she conducted several 12-week songwriting programmes for small groups of abused women. Due to the nature of this project, Day is able to share detailed notes of the various stages involved in composing and refining the songs so the reader can view the evolving product at different points over the 12-week programmes. An important aspect of Day's method is her emphasis on the rehearsing and recording as being integral to the process and explains how these women respond to this process.

For many years now, Randi Rolvsjord has included songwriting as part of her clinical practice in psychiatry. In her chapter, she describes a songwriting approach with patients who have mental health problems as understood within a resource-oriented framework. Such a philosophical approach to music therapy is the topic of her current doctoral studies at Aalborg University, Denmark. In outlining her method, Rolvsjord describes the care and consideration she gives to selecting musical form. In particular, she discusses the use of verse–refrain structures, the use of bridges and tags, and the value in selecting Norwegian folk song forms to facilitate the songwriting process.

Having recently completed a thematic analysis of songs composed by clients within therapy (Baker, Kennelly and Tamplin in press[a], in press[b]), Felicity Baker, Jeanette Kennelly and Jeanette Tamplin describe the role of songwriting in exploring identity change and sense of self-concept following traumatic brain injury (TBI). The difficulties experienced by TBI patients are clearly explained and exemplified, which adds significantly to an understanding of the method. The songwriting method and techniques used by these authors such as 'fill-in-the-blank', 'song parody' and 'song collage technique' are very well defined in this chapter, and provide a clear model.

Felicity Baker also writes on songwriting with people with traumatic brain injury, but here she concentrates on the functional use of songwriting with this population where the intervention is specifically applied to address acquired impairments in pragmatics for functional and developmental skills. Baker's experience is underpinned not only by her long experience in working with the neurological population, but also from her doctoral research. She is very detailed and procedural in explaining the method of writing songs, especially from the perspective of how musical accompaniments and melodies are developed. This chapter explains the process of 'crafting' a song, and as such provides a very important direction on method and technique that enables a student or therapist to apply the model.

Trygve Aasgaard completed a comprehensive and qualitative study on songwriting with paediatric patients in oncology at Aalborg University and has since reported his clinical work (Aasgaard 2000, 2001). In his chapter, he explains the principles of songwriting as he applies it in a hospital for sick children, and in the clinical examples reveals important differences between how this works with younger and older children. A significant aspect in Aasgaard's work is the 'relationship' formed by other members of a child's family to the song, and how it holds a special place for them, as well as sometimes being performed by them. The afterlife of the song is also referred to in this chapter. The case studies here sensitively illustrate the value of the songs as vehicles of expression for some of the most difficult aspects of treatment in oncology.

Emma O'Brien also researched her clinical work for a Masters study at The University of Melbourne (O'Brien 2003), and has been committed to the value of written songs for palliative care patients both in their therapeutic process and for recording and ensuring the lasting life of the song as part of a released CD of songs. She presents a detailed explanation of her method, with notated examples that show exactly the process by which she first draws on the ideas of the patient, then offers musical suggestions, and through this process, crafts a song. The care with which

O'Brien ensures the song always belongs to a client, and that the client has real choice even when not in any way musically trained, is one of the most important methodological aspects of this chapter, which she describes as Guided Songwriting.

Like Derrington, Robert Krout also presents work with teenagers, but in this situation he works with bereaved adolescents and applies his own songs in therapy, which have been pre-composed to meet the very specific needs of this population. He describes a ten-step approach to composing and arranging songs that again provides a very clearly described method that can be applied in therapy. Krout comes with a significant and well-known history and experience of using guitar skills in therapy, and he exemplifies this with examples in his use of songs with teenagers. Group work is also an important feature of this chapter, as Krout focuses on the genre and lyrics that are going to be most relevant and understandable to this age group, and with which they will be able to identify. Krout also refers to the more technical aspects of equipment that is useful in this work.

The chapter by Dileo and Magill provides a unique perspective on songwriting by drawing attention to the multicultural considerations one might encounter when writing songs together with oncology and hospice patients. From a solid theoretical frame, these experienced clinicians/researchers explore songwriting with consideration given to 'collectivist' versus 'individualist' views on world culture and how these influence the songwriting process and the song product. This chapter provides an overview of different multicultural song forms with clear illustrations of rhythmic patterns, melodic styles, harmonic progressions and stanza structures that suit a variety of different non-Western song forms. While this chapter focuses on oncology and hospice patients from varied cultural backgrounds, the principles and information they detail are useful for clinicians working with other multicultural client groups.

The final chapter by Wigram looks at the similarities and differences between the different methods of songwriting that have been described by the contributors. How different practitioners approach this form of intervention with methods that range on a spectrum from broad guiding principles to staged protocols is examined to summarize material that was intended to mark out this text as one which reports method and technique. The relevance of the style of approach related to the needs of differing populations is considered and a review of musical song styles used by contributors is included. Finally, a flexible generic method is outlined that can act as a framework for songwriting in music therapy.

1

Improvised Songs and Stories in Music Therapy Diagnostic Assessments at a Unit for Child and Family Psychiatry

A Music Therapist's and a Psychotherapist's Perspective

Amelia Oldfield and Christine Franke

This chapter presents an opportunity to reflect on both the musical and the verbal content of the improvised songs and stories that are used as part of the music therapy diagnostic assessments at the Croft Unit for Child and Family Psychiatry. The verbal content of the songs and stories the children told in therapy are fascinating to the authors and presents challenges to the potential interpretation and use of this material. The music therapist also wanted to explore how the verbalizations related to and were influenced by the music-making.

As part of her doctoral research into how children on the Autistic Spectrum express, process and regulate emotions, the psychotherapist, Christine Franke, had observed a number of videos of Amelia Oldfield and Emma Davies' music therapy sessions at the Croft Unit. The text of the children's stories had been transcribed by the psychotherapist and she also documented her clinical observations. Through their discussions, the music therapist frequently gained new insights into the possible meanings of the verbal content from the psychotherapist's more psychodynamic interpretations. The authors therefore decided to write this chapter together, drawing material from videos of music therapy sessions which the psychotherapist had observed and analysed. Songs and stories from five children Amelia

Oldfield assessed and two children Emma Davies assessed are included in this account.

In this chapter, the procedures used by the music therapists to facilitate the creation of these improvised songs with individual children will be described in detail. The role of the music, the words and the non-verbal communication will be explored in depth. The ways in which the improvised songs enable both the music therapists and the psychotherapist to gain a better understanding of the child's emotional world, ways of thinking and general strengths and difficulties will be explained. These new insights often influence the team diagnosis given to the child during admission to the unit.

Throughout the chapter, children's improvised songs and stories are referred to and analysed. To preserve confidentiality, the names of the children and some of the verbal content of the stories have been changed.

This chapter will introduce readers to the use of improvised songs and stories as part of a diagnostic process. Although some children respond more to one aspect of these improvisations than others, each child's creation is unique, and the stories are one-off events rather than on-going processes that evolve over time. For this reason it has not been possible to categorize the information in this chapter in table form. Instead we have used headings to try to show that various aspects of the improvised songs or stories will provide the most interesting diagnostic information for individual children.

The Croft Unit for Child and Family Psychiatry

The Croft Unit is a psychiatric assessment centre for children up to the age of 13 and their families. There are usually no more than eight children attending at the Croft at any one time, with a wide range of disorders such as autistic spectrum disorder, Tourette Syndrome or eating disorders. Some families are admitted residentially, or on a daily basis, ranging from four weeks to three to four months. During the day the children attend the unit school in the morning. In the afternoon they attend various groups, such as social skills, art and recreation groups which are run by the unit's staff.

Staff on the unit include: psychiatrists, a family therapist, specialist nurses, a teacher, classroom assistants, health care assistants, clinical psychologists and music therapists. Social workers, health visitors and the teachers involved with the children outside the unit work closely with staff on the unit.

The strengths and difficulties of the children and the families admitted to the Croft are evaluated in different ways. The clinical psychologist carries out a number of psychological tests such as the Parenting Stress Index (Abidin 1995) as well as other cognitive or developmental tests on the children such as the Wechsler Intelligence Scale for Children (Wechsler 1992). Sometimes special questionnaires are devised by the clinical psychologist for different members of staff on the unit to complete, particularly when the team are trying to observe and understand children's or families' difficulties which occur in unpredictable and erratic ways. Specially trained staff carry out the Autism Diagnostic Observation Schedule (ADOS) and the Autism Diagnostic Interview (ADI) (Lord *et al*. 1989 and Dilavore, Rutter and Lord 1995).

The first author has been working as a music therapist at the Croft Unit for Child and Family Psychiatry for 17 years. Initially, the unit admitted children and families for up to 18 months but in the past ten years the work on the unit has focused more clearly on assessments and short-term treatment. Children and families are now routinely admitted for four-week assessments and may then be treated for up to three months with the occasional child or family staying on for six months. As a result of this shift in focus, the music therapist developed some specific Music Therapy Diagnostic Assessments (MTDAs) which assist the team in determining the children's strengths and difficulties.

During the past five years Oldfield set up a PhD research investigation comparing the MTDAs with the ADOS (Oldfield 2004). The study indicated that the MTDAs were serving a useful and distinct purpose in helping the psychiatric team to diagnose children. The MTDAs are now routinely used by both music therapists working at the Croft, and have now become an established part of the diagnostic process at the Croft.

The Music Therapy Diagnostic Assessments

The MTDAs consist of two half-hour sessions, which usually occur at the same time and on the same day of the week over two consecutive weeks. A time will be arranged for two music therapy assessment sessions and the child will be informed about the sessions in a morning meeting when the child's timetable for that day is explained. The music therapist will introduce herself to the child when she goes to collect him or her and they may 'chat' informally as they walk to the music therapy room.

The purpose of the music therapy diagnostic assessments

The overall purpose of these assessments is to use a different medium (music-making) to help the team in assessing children's strengths and difficulties. The questions the Croft team is seeking to answer will vary tremendously depending on each child and it is therefore difficult to outline the general purpose of the assessments. However, experience and research (Oldfield 2004) have shown that music therapy diagnostic assessments are particularly effective at evaluating children's non-verbal communication skills. Further, the music-making often produces heightened states of arousal in the children which enable the therapist to evaluate how they operate when they are very involved and engaged. Because of this heightened state of arousal children's tics or repetitive ritualistic behaviours are often more frequent in music therapy diagnostic assessments. The music therapist can then observe and try to understand these behaviours in the children.

Music-making often allows the therapist to observe emotional responses or the lack of emotional responses in the children, in ways that may be different from the children's reactions in other non-musical settings. The verbal content of the songs and stories can give insight into new aspects of the children's inner world and also into how children regulate and deal with their emotions.

The music therapist feeds back her findings to the team in weekly management meetings. As there is not enough time to report back on all the strengths and difficulties she will have observed in a child arising from the MTDA, the music therapist will select those pieces of information which seem to shed a new or different light on the child's abilities and difficulties. It is this new view of the child which is often of interest to the team. Occasionally, the music therapist's observations will confirm what the rest of the team are saying, in which case the music therapist will give a few examples of events which support the opinion of her colleagues.

The room / equipment

The room is equipped with a piano, an electric organ, several guitars, and a wide range of simple percussion and wind instruments. There are also two small violins and the music therapist uses her own clarinet. All the instruments are laid out on shelves or stand near the wall and are accessible to the children.

Two small chairs (child size) stand facing one another a little distance from the instruments. Two bigger chairs are in front of the piano. The floor is carpeted and there are a few pictures on the wall: drawings and collages obviously done by children. There is no other furniture except some more stacked up children's chairs. The room is friendly and spacious but has few distractions. The open shelves covered with instruments invite the child to take an interest in music-making. But there is also a sense of tidiness and organization conveyed by the carefully set out chairs.

Structure of the session

The following is a description of the format which is normally used. However, there will always be exceptions and the music therapist tries to be flexible to meet the needs of each child so that she can create the optimum situation and setting to evaluate a child's strengths and weaknesses.

First, the child is invited to sit down on a chair facing the music therapist. The music therapist says something like 'here's a chair for you and I'll sit here', usually gesturing as she speaks. The session then begins with a 'hello song' that the music therapist sings to the child incorporating the child's name and accompanying herself by playing chords on the guitar. The session ends with a percussion duet on the bongo drums where the music therapist sings 'good bye' and makes a clear ending. At some point, either at the beginning or at the end of the session (or as the music therapist and the child are walking to or from the music therapy room), the music therapist explains that they will be having two individual sessions together and reminds the child of the time of the session the following week.

In between the 'hello' and the 'good bye', the music therapist explains that they will take turns to choose what to do together. This structure gives the children the freedom to choose and make their own decisions but also allows the therapist to ensure she can implement the tasks she has prepared. If the process of choosing is too difficult or painful, the child can relax at the times when the music therapist provides him or her with her own choices and perhaps a reassuring structure. From the point of view of assessing the child's strengths and weaknesses, the music therapist can find out a great deal from the ways in which the child chooses instruments and activities in music therapy sessions.

As one of 'her' choices the music therapist chooses improvised songs/stories. These will now be examined in more depth.

Improvised stories and songs

As with most aspects of Oldfield's music therapy work, the method of facilitating the creation of improvised stories and songs evolved through her music therapy practice, where every child's song or story in some way informed and influenced the way she implemented the method with subsequent children. Gradually, a system and some theoretical ideas have evolved, but these ideas will continue to change and grow as the work continues. This is why the authors have chosen to describe the work and case studies first and reflect on the evolving methodology later in this chapter.

Case example: Allan's story

Allan is aged 12 and has a diagnosis of autistic spectrum disorder. He was admitted because he was having violent outbursts, had been excluded from school and was struggling at home, often being aggressive towards his mother. He had engaged freely in the musical dialogues with the music therapist (Amelia Oldfield) in the session before the story was suggested. As soon as the therapist sings 'once upon a time there was a…' he starts playing and singing freely. His singing style matches the diatonic notes he plays on the bass xylophone and fits in with the therapist's melodic line. He sings about a troll called 'Albert' and a Mummy troll. Albert brought some goggles and they went swimming. At this point the therapist says: '…and suddenly they saw a crocodile…what happened?' Allan continues playing but doesn't sing or say anything… The therapist encourages a response by playing unresolved cadences and questioning phrases. Suddenly Allan starts chanting an unconnected 'rap': 'Hey, baby, yea, I'm playing today, one two three, I'm playing today…' The therapist now verbally says: '…but what happened to the trolls in the story when the crocodile came?' …exasperated, Allan says: 'The crocodile exploded…and that was the end of the story.'

The music therapist was impressed with Allan's creativity and by his ability to listen to her musical ideas as well as initiate his own ideas. She found herself enjoying making music with Allan and felt that he was communicative through his playing. However, he was not willing to incorporate her verbal suggestions into the story. The psychotherapist pointed out that he might also have suddenly ended the story because he wanted to avoid thinking about conflicts and be unwilling to explore violence in a story. For the Croft team it was important to find out that Allan could be more communicative in a reciprocal way when he was using a non-verbal form of exchange than when he was talking. This observation contributed towards the Croft suggested diagnosis that he was on the milder end of the autistic spectrum. It was also useful to find out that he was purposefully shying away from talking about violence or aggression, indicating that he was in some way aware of these difficulties in his life, but unwilling to talk or think about them at the moment.

General description

During one of the music therapist's choices she places a number of large instruments such as the drum, the metallophone and the wind chimes in front of the child and then goes to the piano. Before starting to play, she says something like 'this is my choice and I'm going to choose for us to make up a story together'. They start playing together freely and then the music therapist says: 'Let's make up a story…once upon a time there was a…' In many cases the child will complete the sentence and say '…a dog!' (for example). They improvise music together and the music therapist might say '…where did the dog go?' and the story evolves, accompanied by musical improvisations.

It is clear from the vignette on the previous page that the musical components, the non-verbal communication and the verbal content of the story are all interrelated aspects of the improvised songs and stories. Nevertheless, an attempt will now be made to examine each of these different elements, and try to explore and explain the variety of ways in which both the child and the therapist use the musical components, the non-verbal communication and the verbal content of the songs and the stories and how the music therapist facilitates the process.

The musical components

THE THERAPIST'S MUSIC

The therapist will usually start by giving the child a large wooden bass xylophone and a cymbal and sit down at the piano explaining that they will tell a story together. The xylophone is chosen because it is a large appealing-looking instrument, which most children want to try out. It is solid, but not very loud, so it is possible to hear the song or story at the same time as the instrument is played. The cymbal is usually offered with the wooden xylophone, to allow for loud 'crashes' and a contrasting sound. However, if the child has already used these instruments a lot in the music therapy diagnostic assessment, other instruments such as the metallophone and the drum may be chosen instead.

To begin with, the therapist usually creates a 'bland' atmosphere by playing 'neutral' music to attempt to create a reassuring atmosphere without associations. If the child starts playing immediately, the therapist's introduction will be influenced by that child's playing – she might match the child's rhythm, for example, or pick up on a characteristic short melodic phrase. If the child does not play, the therapist might be influenced by the child's posture or expression, or by the style of improvising which has preceded the improvised song. When the child has been offered a diatonic xylophone with no sharps or flats the music therapist will usually play in C major, using simple, predictable 'non-confrontative' IV (subdominant), V (dominant) and I (tonic) type chord sequences, in order to fit in with, and not clash with, the child's improvising. At this point the music therapist is careful not to play well-known tunes or phrases that might have specific associations for the child. The therapist will sing in a similar musical style, using the following words 'once upon a time, there was a…', pausing in an expectant way after the 'was a…' to encourage an answer from the child. An example of a typical opening musical phrase is illustrated in Figure 1.1.

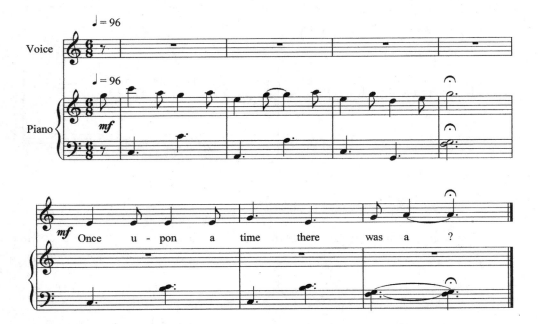

Figure 1.1 'Open' C major introduction

Some children will immediately play music with the therapist and a musical interlude may then precede the story-telling. Other children will be encouraged to engage by the therapist's opening words to the story and the therapist will then match her accompaniment to the child's playing at the same time as starting the story.

Once the story gets going, the therapist's musical accompaniment can either support or interrupt the storyline. The therapist can support the story musically by providing appropriate sound effects such as a fast chromatic scale to illustrate running (Figure 1.2)…:

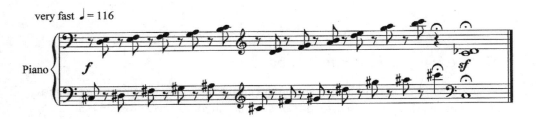

Figure 1.2 Sound effects for a chase

...a sudden two-handed clashing loud chord at the bottom of the piano for a crash; spooky, repeated chromatic phrases to increase tension (Figure 1.3)...:

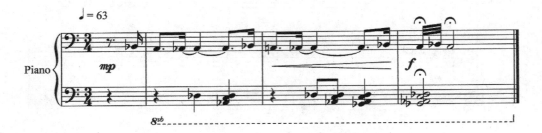

Figure 1.3 'Spooky moment'

...or slow, quiet, pentatonic phrases at the top of the keyboard to illustrate peaceful sleep (Figure 1.4):

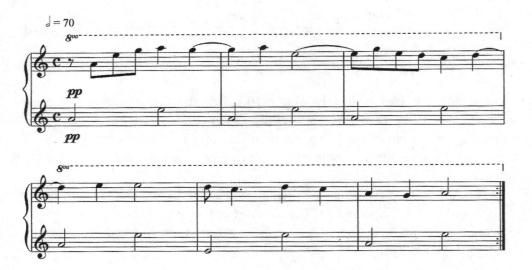

Figure 1.4 'Sleepy music'

Case example: Emanuel's song

Emanuel, who is ten and has attention deficit disorder, behaviour problems and possible autistic spectrum disorder or specific language problems, sings about a queen called 'Tracey'. The music therapist (Amelia Oldfield) supports this idea by playing the opening chords to 'God save the queen'. Encouraged, Emanuel adds that she is the most beautiful queen in the world and that she has a little dog called Candy, who is the most beautiful dog in the world. Emanuel then loses the thread a little, continues singing with enthusiasm but uses unconnected words which are difficult to decipher. The therapist gives him time by interacting with him musically. She is careful not to probe about the meaning of Emanuel's words as she knows that he is sensitive about his language difficulties and can easily be discouraged. In order to 'bring him back' after a few minutes of playing together, she suddenly changes to a faster, more dynamic, rhythmic style of playing. He responds by also playing more energetically and stops his aimless verbalizing. The therapist is then able to ask him more about the queen in the story. He answers that she had four children who end up being his siblings and himself. They all go to the park and when the therapist inserts a cat into the story, Candy the dog 'just leaves the cat alone and smiles at her'. In this story, the musical accompaniment has enabled Emanuel to be supported and then re-engaged in his story-telling. The music therapist gets the impression that she is more able to influence Emanuel through her musical ideas and challenges than through her verbal suggestions, which don't change the storyline in any way.

The therapist may 'interrupt' by suddenly stopping, changing style, inserting a clashing chord, or changing tempo or dynamics. Sometimes the therapist will provide longer musical interludes in order to give a child time and space to think about and reflect upon an issue. Similarly, a verbal phrase in the story may be repeated in a variety of musical ways in order to give particular words emphasis, or to give the child time to think about the sequel.

THE CHILD'S MUSIC

Each child's music is unique, but there are some patterns that seem to emerge regarding the ways in which the children use the music.

For many children it seems to be the music-making that initially draws them into the shared activity and then enables them to create stories and songs. Some children immediately start singing as soon as the therapist sings. Like Emanuel, children are often uninhibited musically but more stuck verbally, playing and/or singing freely but either not speaking at all or producing unconnected words.

Styles of singing will vary, from choirboy voices to 'rock' or 'rap', from plainsong to operatic type vibrato or recitative. Sometimes children will 'become' a particular favourite pop singer, or suddenly switch from one style to another in the same way that Allan suddenly lapsed into a rap to avoid incorporating the music therapist's crocodile into his story. Some children will choose to speak rather than sing.

Many children use patterns in their playing and their singing, either repeated rhythmic patterns such as the 'shave and a haircut today' rhythm (Figure 1.5), or short repeated melody lines.

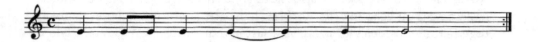

Figure 1.5 'Shave and a haircut today' rhythm

Sometimes the children lose themselves in these musical repetitions and forget about the storyline altogether. Occasionally children will become diverted from the storyline by wanting to produce a particular tune or recreate a special sound effect. The therapist can gently attempt to re-engage the child in the story-telling and observe how easy or difficult this might be for the child.

Case example: Henry's song

Henry, aged six, has a diagnosis of autistic spectrum disorder. He immediately starts vocalizing as soon as the music therapist (Emma Davies) starts singing. Some words are included in his vocalizations, but it appears that it is the singing rather than the verbal content which is the focus of his attention. He sings in a clear voice, with some vibrato, matching the diatonic phrases on the bass xylophone and the piano. His spontaneous and creative singing, which shows that he is both listening to the music therapist and able to initiate his own musical ideas, is in stark contrast to the story which he eventually tells. He wants to tell the story of the three pigs. When the therapist encourages him to tell a 'new' story, he compromises by agreeing to a story about one pig. While he continues to play and sing freely, he reminds the therapist that the pig is called 'Jack' and is not called 'Henry', and that the wolf is called 'Violin' (a violin lies on a shelf in front of him). The words he uses must be clear and well defined. The verbal exchanges with Emma in the story remain rather unimaginative, but at the same time Henry can be remarkably creative and fluid in his musical exchanges with the music therapist, spontaneously both matching and initiating melodic and rhythmic phrases.

At times Henry's movements are quite dramatic and he makes large theatrical gestures before producing flurries of notes on the bass xylophone. At other times he fiddles with the beaters. When the wolf bites the pig's head, Henry taps his own head with the beaters, again wanting to make the words in the story clear and concrete.

The most striking thing about Henry's story is in his means of engagement and presentation. Verbally he seeks control, describes some violent actions and is concerned about names of characters, possibly confused about his own identity. However, musically, he is very free and fluid and can both listen and initiate ideas. At the weekly management meeting the team were surprised to learn how creative and spontaneous Henry could be in his non-verbal interactions. The consultant psychiatrist wondered whether it might be appropriate to question his diagnosis of 'classical' autism in favour of a less severe type of autism.

Allan, Emanuel and Henry all seemed more at ease with the non-verbal aspects of communication in the stories than with the verbal exchanges. We will now look in more depth at these non-verbal exchanges and at what the therapist can learn about a child through the non-verbal aspects of improvised songs and stories.

Case example: Joe

Joe, aged 8 with severe attachment disorder, initially wouldn't play the instruments and couldn't think of anything to say in the story. The music therapist (Amelia Oldfield) played a rhythmic tune in a major key and Joe started laughing hysterically, swaying in his chair and saying 'I always laugh when I'm happy'. As she watched Joe, the therapist felt a wave of desperation and sadness, and recognized that she was possibly picking up Joe's feelings, although what he was saying and doing were the opposite to what she thought he was experiencing. A very banal story about a boy going to a park and playing on the swings then evolved. However, at one point the sudden appearance of a fox (suggested by the therapist) led to Joe suddenly and briefly playing the cymbal very loudly and angrily. The therapist didn't feel that this playing was related to the storyline or the musical accompaniment, but rather to Joe's inner turmoil. Perhaps the fact that he allowed himself albeit briefly to express his anguish was related to the fact that the therapist had picked up some of his non-verbal signals. The music therapist was clearly experiencing counter-transference here. It is important for her to be aware of this process and to be sure that the feeling is not hers in the first place but something that belongs to the child, but is yet unexpressed.

Non-verbal communication

After the instruments have been put in front of the child and the therapist has sat down at the piano, started playing and said 'let's tell a story…', the therapist will take cues from the child to decide how to proceed. If the child immediately engages in the story-telling, then the verbal content will influence the therapist. If the child engages in music-making or singing as Henry and Allan did, then the therapist will 'answer' these musical suggestions. However, in many cases the child may be silent or playing in a very vague way, so the therapist looks at the child's body language and facial expression, and also takes note of how the child is making her 'feel'. In the vignette on the next page, for example, there was a clear discrepancy between what the child was saying and what the therapist was feeling.

Sometimes a child's non-verbal communication is much more obvious. Boredom may be expressed by lying on the xylophone, for example. Many children with attention deficit disorder will struggle to focus and the therapist may clear the room of distracting objects or make sure that not too many instruments are available at once. Children with conduct disorder may seek to intimidate the therapist, and find out where the boundaries of what is permitted lie. Often a slow, bored tone of voice devoid of emotion can help diffuse threats, and it may be helpful to explain clearly, in a non-confrontational way, what is and is not acceptable. At other times it may be helpful to divert the child, such as through a surprising change in the music. Again it is not so much the verbal content that is important but the way in which the verbal responses are given.

In many of the children's stories, it is not so much what is said but rather what is not said, or the disconnected or unimaginative aspect of the story which is revealing. A child may, for example, be reluctant to deviate from a familiar well-known story. This could be because the child has no confidence in his or her ability to create a story, or it could be that the child is frightened of 'losing control'. In other cases a child might suddenly stop a story when material comes up that the child does not wish to consider in any way. This is illustrated in Leon's story:

Case example: Leon's story

Leon was aged five and diagnosed as having autistic spectrum disorder. His story went like this:

> Once there was a black cow…her name was Leon. (And where did she go?) The farmyard where she met a lady called Lorna Hex. (Leon insists on the 'Hex' being used.) Leon the black cow and Lorna Hex go to the beach and there is a man there and they play with a ball.

The music therapist (Amelia Oldfield) takes the story on and becomes quite excited in her telling that 'as they play the water comes nearer and nearer and what happens?' 'They drown,' says Leon. 'Just like that?' asks the therapist. 'Yea,' Leon replies. She repeats this last part of the story and then asks Leon if they should make an ending. 'Let's count to four.' They do, and end together.

Leon's story is relatively unimaginative. He uses his own name and although the cow may have some meaning to him this seems not so likely. The name Lorna Hex seems to be a person he knows and one imagines he likes as he insists on the full title being given. The story is told in early summer, so the beach will probably have been talked about at home or at school. When the therapist takes the story over, both musically by energetic and excited playing and also in adding to the story, Leon stops the story: 'they both drown'. It was said with a finality. This might indicate that Leon deals with emotional situations by blotting them out rather than confronting them.

Leon was a child whom the psychotherapist had observed in other settings apart from during the improvised story. She was therefore able to note that there was a pattern emerging that whenever he was over-stimulated or the level of emotional arousal was too hard for him to process he seemed to 'disconnect' from contact. During the story there were times when he fidgeted or appeared to ignore the music therapist's suggestions. So in this story, the drowning of both the characters is in keeping with the other observations of his dealing with emotional events: there is no thought or processing – just a cessation.

Verbal content of the songs and the stories

THE THERAPIST'S VERBAL CONTENT

After the introduction, the therapist might encourage a child to get going by saying or singing 'was it a dog or a cat?' for example. The therapist will often suggest familiar domestic animals because many children will be interested in these animals and will easily make associations, which will produce imaginative ideas. Sometimes the therapist might start the story with 'once upon a time there was a…(and if the child says nothing)…a boy'. But introducing people rather than animals can more easily lead to an account of something that happened rather than a 'new' story, which is what is being aimed at. If the child starts a well-known story such as 'Once upon a time there were three bears…' the therapist might attempt to change things a little by saying something like: '…and they lived in a castle with a magician…' In a similar way children can get stuck in repetitive sequences and, if the therapist feels that there is no more to be gained or learnt from these repetitions, she might purposely interrupt or try to help the child change direction. The therapist could introduce a change by making a 'new' verbal contribution or by making a significant musical change (e.g. a sudden change of volume, rhythm or style).

In many cases, but particularly if the child has not brought any confrontation into the story, the therapist might attempt to incorporate an element of adversity such as a crocodile, a wolf or a monster. This increases the emotional tone of the story and allows the therapist to observe how the child deals with confrontation.

The therapist often chooses elements to bring into the stories because of specific previous knowledge of a child's likes/dislikes or particular strengths or difficulties. Many children on the autistic spectrum have favourite topics such as 'aliens' or 'turtles' and the therapist may introduce an 'alien' or a 'turtle' in order to engage and interest a child. Conversely, she may take care to avoid 'aliens' or 'turtles' if she feels these topics will mean that the child becomes isolated in 'set' stories rather than allowing imagination to flow. Other children may be very emotional about their pets, or sensitive about a recent pet's death, so these characters may not be suggested by the therapist unless she feels it would be useful for the child to use the story to talk about these difficulties. In Joe's case, for example, the therapist knew that he was missing his puppy and often became miserable when he thought about his pet. She therefore avoided suggesting a dog or even a cat (which might have reminded him about pets). She also wanted to see whether she could encourage Joe to be creative rather than remaining very banal, so she tried introducing a 'fox' which is a wild and unpredictable creature, but not necessarily frightening or scary.

Often the therapist will want to find out whether a child is prepared to incorporate the therapist's verbal ideas as well as initiate his/her own. Allan and Leon's vignettes, for example, showed that these two children were not prepared to accept the therapist's contributions. It was helpful for the team to find out that these two children found it difficult to accept these types of adult suggestions, even when it was being done in a playful way.

If a child brings violence or conflict into a story, the therapist makes sure that there is an opportunity to resolve the issues if the child chooses to. However, she will not steer the child towards a resolution if this is not what the child wants. It is important for the therapist to be able to allow for an unhappy ending if this is the child's choice.

The overall structure of the songs and stories varies completely from one child to another. Some of the children's stories may be no longer than one or two sentences, while others may last 20 minutes and have a clear beginning, middle and end. Apart from the introductory sentence and suggestions to help 'get things going' the therapist will not seek to guide the structure in any way.

However, the therapist always tries to help the child make a clear ending to the story, supporting the child to find a way to finish in whatever way is accessible to the child. Younger children might go 'one, two, three, finish' (such as Leon), others might say '…and they lived happily ever after' or simply '…and that's the end of the story'.

Case example: Seth's story

Seth, aged 11, had a diagnosis of Asperger's Syndrome. He was a very angry boy who was struggling with aggressive outbursts, which often got him into trouble. He would use these outbursts and verbally hostile attacks to keep people at bay, but was very upset about his behaviour. He and his mother had high expectations of the Croft to be able to 'sort it out' for him. He told the story with the music therapist (Emma Davies) of a tiger called Mr Stripes who went on holiday to swim with the dolphins. Suddenly he saw a crocodile and he ran away. Then he bit off the crocodile's head. The croc was not dead but couldn't get Mr Stripes. The croc got hit by a speed boat and died in the middle of the lake. Mr Stripes got married to Emma the elephant. He got hungry (there was a long pause) and then he ate his wife. 'And how did Mr Stripes feel?' asked the therapist. 'I'm bored.' Mr Stripes got shoved in a mental home and then he came out and he was free.

From her observations of Seth, the psychotherapist felt that the following was a possible interpretation of this story. It seems that Seth can't have what he wants – a fun life and perhaps company and affection. This is seen in the swimming with the dolphins. There is fear of his own destructiveness and anger – this is the crocodile image. There is a part of him that can tackle this in himself, but it is not very effective. This aspect seems too big for his coping self and it is something else (the boat) that 'kills the croc'. The psychotherapist thought that this represented Seth being at the Croft and 'evidenced' his firm belief that the Croft could put this right for him.

Seth's emotional greed, fuelled by his feeling that he never managed to get what he needed and often destroyed what was on offer, is expressed by his choosing a good solid wife who, one can wonder, has many resources, an elephant called Emma. Emma is the name of his music therapist. It was apparent from the way Seth worked with the music therapist that he trusted her and felt secure with her. This could be seen as a differing relationship from Mum who was struggling with Seth's aggressive outbursts and was in quite a desperate state at the time. But Seth is telling us that he is unsure of his ability to keep what he needs – he 'eats his wife'. Seth shows us what happens when he wants something – he destroys what he most needs as he can't control his aggression.

However, Seth seems to know that the problem is his and in his head, hence the need for the 'mental home'. This is how he saw the Croft and his belief that they would sort it out for him.

This story illustrates that Seth could think about himself in metaphor. For the team it was helpful to know that Seth had confidence in the Croft and also that Seth could think in this way. As a result, some doubts were cast on his diagnosis of Asperger's Syndrome.

Case example: Thomas' story

Another revealing story was that told by Thomas. Thomas is aged seven and has previously had a diagnosis of autistic spectrum disorder. He appears quite sociable and asks adults many appropriate questions. He obviously thinks about what he sees and about what is going on. However, he tends to ignore other children and at times seems unaware of events happening around him. Thomas had a small alien figure in his pocket and brought it out as he had his session. The alien would do things that Thomas didn't want to do such as hold the beaters. This was his story:

> Once upon a time there was an alien. (Where did the alien go?) He went to the moon. (Who did he meet?) A dinosaur. (And what did they do together?) They made a pie with a cherry on the top. (What was the alien called?) Alfie. (And what is the dinosaur called?) Bailey.
>
> They went shopping and then they returned to earth to find something to eat. (And what did they eat?) They ate a doggie's bone. Then they went to the playground and met a spider, who was called Cymbal. (What did they all do?) They had a chat and went together to the seesaw. They all went to the forest and met a tiger and ran away.
>
> [The music therapist (Amelia Oldfield) plays in an excited manner.] They got away just in time but one was captured – the spider, Cymbal. But they had a plan – they made a monster and the tiger flew away. (Is that the finish?) The spider was saved and they lived happily.

The psychotherapist suggested that this story could have a meaning for him and that the three characters represented aspects of his own self. Thomas may well have identified himself with both the alien and the dinosaur, Bailey. It feels possible that Thomas has a story about a dinosaur and that it was an isolated and perhaps ostracized creature. The creatures were happy in the 'other world' of the moon as they made a pie with a cherry on the top: there is an ideal feel to this world. But this wasn't enough: they needed more 'food', so they came back to earth – to the 'normal' shared world of others – to go shopping. What Thomas tells us is that the 'food' here is not as special as the pie with the cherry. It is measly food, 'a doggie's bone', that doesn't seem very good for him.

The psychotherapist feels that this is how it may feel to Thomas – he wants to be part of the 'normal world', but finds that his autistic world is more fulfilling, it is less stressful and he can withdraw into it.

They meet a spider called Cymbal – named after the object in front of his eyes. The psychotherapist felt that this represented the part of himself that is vulnerable when he is 'on earth'. The tiger may represent one of two aspects. It may be the hostile feelings of others that he feels threatened by, and that he uses his alien and dinosaur aspects to rescue his spider self. This could be a happy ending of the three characters reunited, but it suggests there could possibly be a return to the ideal world – that is, into an autistic withdrawal. Or the tiger could represent the more protecting, defensive part of himself that looks after his vulnerability when he is 'on earth' and keeps the difficult things away. However, the sad part of this is that the 'autistic triad' seems to regroup, thus suggesting, again, Thomas' pull to an autistic state.

When feeding back to the team it was important to share that Thomas was thinking about his different worlds and at times consciously retreating into autistic behaviours.

THE CHILDREN'S VERBAL CONTENT

In the vignettes involving Allan, Emanuel, Henry, Joe and Leon, the verbal content of the songs and the stories themselves were not as interesting or revealing from a diagnostic point of view as the musical exchanges and the non-verbal interactions. For these children it is aspects such as the ways in which exchanges take place, how much control a child feels he/she needs to have, or the lack of verbal coherence or exchange which are interesting rather than the actual words used.

Many children, however, do become involved in the storylines themselves and through their stories or songs reveal aspects of themselves, which may enable the team to understand them better (see the vignettes involving Seth and Thomas).

Reflections

This chapter has discussed various aspects of improvised songs and stories which form an important part of the music therapy diagnostic assessments at the Croft.

The particular value of improvised songs and stories

Although spontaneous story-telling could be assessed without the improvised music-making, the instrument-playing and singing will often motivate a child and fuel his or her imagination. Acting out the story on the instruments makes the story more exciting and the therapist can improvise on the piano to underline or contain emotions such as excitement, fear or happiness.

The fact that music happens in time, and that musical phrases can be organized to have predictable lengths with endings that can be anticipated, will reassure children and enable some children to relax sufficiently to allow creativity.

Through the improvised music-making, the therapist and the child can be 'equals' as they are both making music freely without reference to a coded language with which the therapist may be more at ease than the child. Some children, however, will not choose to be 'equal' and will really enjoy the fact that they can 'control' the therapist through the improvised songs or stories. The therapist can support and echo these children's stories, giving the child the sense of being listened to and heard. For children who struggle to make decisions and speak up for themselves, the therapist can provide the basic storyline, perhaps limiting the child's decisions to a choice of two items. For the hesitant child, the therapist can provide musical 'padding' to give time for thought processing and decision-making. For the impulsive, 'fast' child, the musical accompaniment can be limited to the odd supportive chord.

The playful aspect of the musical interaction will also appeal to many children who may react to dramatic interchange rather than to verbal exchanges.

In many ways the reasons why these improvised musical stories appeal to children are similar to the general reasons why music therapy assessments are effective with this client group (Oldfield 2000, 2004). The musical exchange, the many aspects of non-verbal communication and the verbal content of the stories combine to provide interesting and often different pictures of the children being diagnosed at the Croft.

The purpose of the improvised songs and stories within the MTDA

The particular value of these songs and stories within the MTDA is that they allow the music therapist to evaluate how a child interacts verbally as well as non-verbally. The rest of the MTDA focuses mainly on non-verbal musical reactions, so in the improvised songs and stories the way the child uses (or fails to use) words or vocalizations will reveal new information.

Sometimes it is not so much the words themselves that are interesting as the relationship between the words and the music-making. The way in which a child switches from verbal to non-verbal types of communication might be particularly striking, or the discrepancy between a child's ability to communicate non-verbally and their ability to communicate through language could be significant.

Interpreting the verbal content of the stories

As a psychoanalytic psychotherapist, Franke believes in the basis of psychoanalysis which suggests that, given a blank sheet, we will express something of ourself, of our internal world as well as our relationships and difficulties in the external world. She thinks that the stories and songs invented in the MTDA are a form of free association.

The procedure of free association is fundamental to psychoanalytic technique as an expression of a spontaneous self-expression. The 'free' in free association does not imply an absence of determination as the first goal is the elimination of the voluntary selection of thoughts. Freud saw this, in the ideas of his second topography, as the incapacity of the second censorship between the conscious and the pre-conscious leading to the unconscious being revealed (Laplanche and Pontalis 1973).

Later, free association was developed by Melanie Klein for her work with children (Klein 1932). Over time she used her observations of children playing with their toys and realized that the elements of the play were manifestations, not solely of the unconscious, but of internal dramas, fantasies, states of mind and parts of the self.

Although some aspects of the interpretations made of the children's songs and stories may be based on traditional aspects of free association, it must be remembered that the meanings of these interpretations depend very much on each individual child's thought processes. For example in Thomas' story the pie with the cherry on the top might, in 'Kleinian' terms, have been seen as the breast. However, it was felt that, for Thomas, it merely represented 'an ideal situation'.

Studying the improvised songs and stories of the children at the Croft has led the psychotherapist to conclude, not surprisingly, that the greater the degree of autism, the less the child appears to show any sense of an internal world. Autistic children, it is suggested, live very much in the surface of the 'here and now' and experience social situations as isolated pictures (Vermeulen 2001).

The sort of stories the children tell and the way they use their imagination in the stories and songs will give the therapist some idea of the child's inner world and of how they form relationships with others.

When to use or not use improvised songs and stories

Most children at the Croft have enjoyed taking part in the improvised songs and stories, and their stories and songs have helped those working with them to understand a little more about the children. However, there have been some occasions when the music therapist has chosen not to use these improvised songs or stories. These occasions have been when a child had obvious problems with speaking, such as children who were selective mutes, had very poor language skills or children who spoke very little or not at all and would have been at a total loss when asked to 'tell a story'. On another occasion the music therapist elected not to introduce the improvised story with a child who had very obsessional language. She felt that she had more chance of a spontaneous exchange through a totally non-verbal medium than by introducing language, which she suspected would be meaningless and would very quickly become totally centred around the child's customary obsessions. Extracting verbal suggestions from children who have a very poor sense of self can also sometimes be a very difficult process and in some cases is too traumatic for the children to maintain an interest in the music-making process.

Nevertheless, it is rare that the improvised songs or stories cannot be adapted in some way to enable the child to combine verbal contributions with musical suggestions in some way which will both maintain the child's interest and help the therapist to understand something more about that child.

Conclusion

The authors have both learnt a great deal from analysing these songs/stories together. Amongst other things, the music therapist has learnt how children may be revealing sides of their inner world, or that children are unable or unwilling to enter into their inner world in any way. The psychotherapist has become aware of the discrepancy that often exists between a child's creative musical interactions and that same child's refusal to engage in meaningful verbal exchanges. The authors will continue to work together. A future project might be to write a more detailed article on one child's improvised story, analysing all the musical content, the non-verbal components of the exchanges as well as the verbal content.

2

You Ask Me Why I'm Singing

Song-creating with Children at a Child and Family Psychiatric Unit

Emma Davies

I've spent my life watching sky and sea change colour
Hypnotised by the beauty of it all
And you ask me why I'm singing
Well it is good for me, it can be good for you

(From *Songs from the Rain* by Hothouse Flowers)

Introduction

Over the last couple of years I have found that songwriting or song-creating has played an increasingly important part of my music therapy work with children. It has had a positive impact not only on the children, but also on their families, peers and other people involved in their care. The aim of this chapter is to highlight how beneficial and relevant this way of working can be and to discuss the methods and ideas that work particularly well with this client group. I will briefly describe the pathology and unique characteristics of this population and explore how this influences the way I approach this work. I will then show how my method is put into practice and illustrate this with two case examples.

The process of creating and singing songs seems to come quite naturally to some children experiencing emotional and communication difficulties, especially those who are approaching adolescence. For many – if not most – adolescence can be a very intense and confusing time of life and it can be difficult to share these emotions. Many children also discover music at this point in their lives and find that certain songs seem to express something of the confusions of emotions they are experiencing. In a recent interview, the 19-year-old Canadian singer Avril Lavigne said:

> Most of my songs are kind of like written when I'm confused, when I'm going through stuff, you know… I think it also has to do with my age, being a teenager – I'm emotional all the time. (Lavigne 2004)

Adolescents may have started to form stylistic preferences and have even tried to emulate their favourite singers. As the comedian Bill Cosby put it: 'By the time a child is eight or nine, he has developed a passion for his own music that is even stronger than his passions for procrastination and weird clothes' (Cosby 1988, p.11). I see it as my role to develop children's relationship with music.

In my experience as a music therapist I have observed that many children who are usually unable to express themselves verbally feel able to do so through the medium of song. Creating a song can help children externalize some of the issues that they are facing and, in the process, give their difficulties a more manageable form. In one of my case examples I discuss how a young adolescent who found it very difficult to talk about his problems, especially to his mother, was able to sing about them. Certainly for some children it seems more socially acceptable, and perhaps less threatening, to channel their emotions into this creative form. Some have even found that writing their own songs gained them the attention and respect of their peers, as discussed in my other case example. The process therefore can help increase children's self-confidence and self-esteem, provide them with a creative way to express themselves, and help them discover a tool that they will, it is hoped, continue to use beyond the music therapy space.

The setting

The children I work with attend the Croft Unit for Child and Family Psychiatry in Cambridge, where I have been based since 2000. The Croft is an inpatient psychiatric unit which provides assessment, diagnostic and treatment work for children up to the age of 13. Many of the children admitted have complex emotional, behavioural or developmental disorders, including severe conduct disorders, attachment disorders, bipolar disorders, psychosomatic illnesses, eating disorders and neurodevelopment disorders, such as autistic spectrum disorder and Asperger's Syndrome. Children are admitted residentially with their families. This enables the multidisciplinary team to gain a global view of the difficulties and to understand the child within the context of his/her family. Support, whether it is by a formal diagnosis or other interventions, is then provided.

Many of the children who have complex emotional and behavioural difficulties find it very difficult to express themselves verbally and to find a voice within their families or peer groups. Some children will have spent a great deal of time being tested and assessed by many professionals, usually focusing on their weaknesses. They may have become locked in a negative cycle of failure and frustration resulting in low self-esteem and a lack of motivation to give anything a try. They may also find it difficult to trust and relate to others. Some desperately need an outlet to express themselves and to be heard but may find conventional ways of doing so difficult.

It is important to take these aspects, as well as others such as age, sex, background and culture, into consideration when working with these children as they will have an impact on how the music therapy develops. For example, working with five- or six-year-olds requires a different approach from working with 12- or 13-year-olds. With the former it might be useful to provide sessions with their families to help them interact and communicate with each other. With the latter, who are approaching adolescence, they may want to gain a sense of independence from their families and explore their own identities. It can also be important to be aware of current fashion, musical and cultural trends in order to create an atmosphere to which they feel they can relate. I often undertake my own research of songs, especially current songs in the charts, so that I have a clear idea of the kind of music that may influence the children's tastes. It is therefore important to have an open-minded and flexible approach.

Method

As each case is unique, it is difficult to identify one method that can be applied to all. Indeed the process should not be formulaic as that would defy the very creative environment it attempts to create. However, there are some ideas and ways of working that have emerged out of my clinical practice which I have found particularly useful in working with this client group.

Creating the right environment

Before the concept of songwriting is introduced (by either the child or me), a secure therapeutic relationship should be developed so that the children feel they can trust me, the situation and the music. They need enough time and encouragement to explore different instruments and realise that they *are* able to achieve something. They also need to feel free to express themselves in whatever way they can. My role at this point is to be 'available' (in a Winnicottian sense) and to listen. Within shared musical improvisations I can respond to their musical ideas and help the child feel heard and responded to. The 'right environment' is therefore created within the here-and-now of improvisation but is also beginning to be established on a more emotional level.

Finding the right time and form

The right time to introduce songwriting varies from child to child and for the different needs and directions of the therapy programme. Sometimes it is to direct a change in the treatment when it is needed. I worked with one child who was a selective mute. Initially I worked hard at helping him to communicate in a non-verbal way through musical improvisations. When he later found his voice, I needed to rethink what music therapy could now offer him. As he had already demonstrated that he was able to use music to express himself and was particularly interested in pop and rap music, I felt that songwriting was a natural progression for him (Carter 2004 – published under my maiden name). In this case, the song we created together came to symbolize the end of music therapy and the child's discharge from the unit.

In other cases, song creations have formed a transitional phase in therapy. Another child with whom I worked, who had an eating disorder, found it very difficult to verbalize her feelings. In music therapy she discovered that she enjoyed the creative aspect of musical composition and began to have a very clear idea of how she wanted to use the sessions. Each week she came with musical motifs that she had worked on at home. As co-composers we worked together, trying out and developing ideas before creating pieces that we then recorded. Although these pieces were not songs in the conventional sense, each one had a title and a clear theme and could perhaps be described as 'songs without words' in a Mendelssohnian sense. Although she was very reluctant to talk directly about the difficulties she was facing, she was, however, able to discuss the ideas and feelings that inspired her to create her pieces. In this case, the process of writing songs enabled a child, who was struggling to communicate, to explore her own way of expressing herself through a medium about which she felt confident. It seemed that she needed to explore a non-verbal way of communicating before feeling ready to move on and make use of verbal therapy.

The idea to create a song can be introduced at various stages in the therapy and can be initiated by the child or the therapist. Some children have a very clear idea of what they want to do, others will need some direction and structure from me. Songs can take on many different forms, such as improvised songs and songs which seem to naturally flow on from improvisations. Others can be formally planned and prepared or based on pre-composed songs or on poems. The level of actual writing varies from case to case. As Trygve Aasgaard explained, in his work with children on an oncology ward,

> I prefer to employ the expressions 'create' or 'make' a song rather than to 'write' a song, because writing is just one (and not even an obligatory) element of the creative process. (Aasgaard 2000, p.72)

Addressing therapeutic aims

In some cases, the songwriting process can play a part in achieving some of the therapeutic goals of the multidisciplinary team. For example, if the children usually find it very difficult to accept others' ideas, it might be important that I encourage them to listen to some of my ideas or make some kind of compromise. Although this may be very difficult for some children, the fact that they are really starting to enjoy the sessions, and feel confident enough about them, can make this issue more manageable and less threatening. Some children need support in tolerating making mistakes and to risk initiating their own ideas for fear of failure. For children with very little self-confidence, initially I have to contribute more actively towards the process until they feel they can work more independently. As the process of song-creating evolves, it is often possible to observe and assess many of the children's difficulties. It can also be a place where children's strengths emerge. Many children are pleasantly surprised and find new self-confidence in being able to produce a song.

Encouraging an interest

As I mentioned earlier, music is something that many children have already discovered before they come to music therapy. They may be aware of which songs are in the charts and want to bring a CD of their favourite song or artist to a session. I see this as an important step as the child is beginning to connect what is occurring in music therapy with their life outside. The fact that they are motivated to bring in their own music is also positive and can often act as a catalyst to thinking about creating their own songs. We listen to the music and begin to talk about it. I might encourage the child to think about what it is about the song that particularly appeals to them, whether it be the lyrics, melodic style, instrumentation or general style of the music. In one case a child brought a video of the film *Titanic* so that we could listen to the theme tune in order to re-create it. The process of re-creating may form an important part of songwriting as we start to think and talk together about the structure of song.

Facilitating song creations

The journey from expressing an interest in songs to actually writing one can begin in many different ways. Some children come to music therapy with a clear idea that they would like to write their own songs. In other cases the idea develops naturally out of shared improvisations. If a child is finding it difficult to verbalize their feelings but they are beginning to communicate through music, I will suggest the idea myself for them to think about.

Generating and brainstorming around a theme

An initial stage to writing a song can be to encourage the child to think of a theme. Some children come to music therapy with a clear idea of what they want to sing about, others need support to find a focus for their ideas. We might write ideas down at the time or, if that is difficult, I suggest they take their time and bring ideas for the next session.

We may have a brainstorming session when we think about the chosen theme and what images or musical ideas it brings up. This part of the process can provide an opportunity for the children to talk about what is on their mind without being directly asked. This can provide insight for the multidisciplinary team which then helps them to think about how best to provide support. Beginning with a theme also provides the opportunity to work towards a manageable goal which in many cases has been set by the child. This can be very important for children who feel they are usually set impossible goals or tasks, for example at school or by medical professionals.

Creating lyrics

Often children are keen to begin by thinking about the lyrics. Some may arrive at the session with lyrics that they have written at home, and sometimes we work on them together. Often I act as the scribe, making suggestions and helping with the structuring of the words when necessary, while the children are busy with the thinking.

Usually I suggest that we work on the idea that a song has a chorus and a number of verses. I explain that the chorus is a good place to start as it often sets the atmosphere and tone of the song. We may think about the positioning of certain words or lines which need to stand out. These may be placed at the end of a verse so that the silence immediately afterwards can be used for dramatic effect. Older children in particular can respond very positively to this more 'academic' way of thinking about music as they may have been introduced to the idea in music lessons at school. Younger children may not yet have an interest in thinking in this way and will want to focus on the actual singing and playing side of songwriting. Often these children respond more to improvised storytelling, as Amelia Oldfield and Christine Franke discuss in their chapter in this book.

Writing lyrics can take some time so we might use a proportion of the session each week for this part. The rest of the session may be spent improvising or exploring different ways of playing instruments.

Writing the music

Sometimes we begin with the music. The child may have remembered a particular musical phrase from their favourite song or from an improvisation we played together. Sometimes words can be spontaneously added to an improvisation and therefore one does not always know where a song improvisation ends and where the making of a song that can be reused begins – improvisations often turn out to become wonderful 'songs' (Aasgaard 2000). They may have heard something from a current pop song, like a guitar riff that they want to use and develop. At this point we might refer back to a CD to gain inspiration. They may want to use a particular instrument for their song and will therefore need some practical help. After this my skills as a composer come into play as I help the child utilize the different musical elements that influence and create a song.

We may think about the general style and mood of the song and how we might create this with different combinations of instruments. If we have the lyrics in front of us, we might start trying out ideas for the vocal part. I encourage the children to look at their words and identify which are the most important ones which might need musical emphasis. I might introduce the technique of word-painting – creating music that attempts to describe the emotion or image of a word or phrase. A simple example of this can be heard in John Dowland's lute song 'Flow, my tears' (Dowland 1600) where the key of A minor and the melodic shape – a sequence of descending minor scales – combine to portray the anguish and melancholic imagery of the text. Just as the key in Dowland's song plays an important part of the whole, so too does the key of the child's song and it is important to think about what impact different keys have. I might play music in different keys and ask them which one best suits their song. We think about the texture of the music and whether there should be lots of different musical lines occurring at the same time or whether it should be simple, perhaps unaccompanied. Other elements, such as rhythm, pulse and harmonic pacing, are also taken into account.

Although all these points are considered we may not always follow a formal process. In many cases decisions are made as part of the creative process as we explore ideas together. However, as the music therapist and 'co-composer' I have these musical techniques 'up my sleeve', which can be accessed when appropriate.

When thinking about the musical role that I should play, I try to ascertain whether it would be more beneficial for me to play an active role or a passive, listening role. In one case I was asked by a child to play a bass line on a guitar for his song. This seemed to give him the support he needed to play his music above it. In some cases I simply listen at first, offering encouragement and praise, waiting for the child to ask me to become more actively involved by offering musical ideas.

Beyond the music therapy room: performance and recording

Often the children ask whether they can video or tape their song. This can be a really valuable part of the process as the song starts to exist, not only in the music room and between ourselves, but outside and among family members and friends. The very act of 'performing' the song in front of a video camera or tape recorder can be a huge achievement for some children who have struggled with low self-confidence for a long time. By recording it they then have something tangible to keep and remind them of their achievement, even after they have left the unit. Sometimes children want to take the recording away to listen to by themselves and to work on new ideas. Sometimes they want to play it to their families and peers or to staff on the unit. This can be a very positive experience as not only do the children gain praise and self-esteem but the 'audience' can begin to see some of the child's talents. This can be an especially meaningful experience for the children's families who, for a long time, may have been focusing on the difficulties. One parent found listening to her son's songs (which he performed live to her) very moving and commented that they helped her to gain a better understanding of his difficulties. Another child was very keen to perform her songs to her sisters. I think this helped them see her in a different light. She became a child with a special talent, rather than the 'sick' child to whom they had become accustomed.

Case example: Ellie's story

This case study of Ellie, a 12-year-old girl, admitted for assessment with a possible diagnosis of bipolar disorder and Asperger's Syndrome, will demonstrate how songwriting was introduced after a long period of therapy and how it played a part in helping her express some of the difficulties she was facing at the time. It also illustrates how the experience impacted on her life outside the sessions.

Ellie suffered from extreme mood swings, ranging from depressive episodes and panic attacks to periods of feeling high and full of wild ideas. At the time she was attending music therapy, her mental state had deteriorated to such an extent that she had not attended school for several months. Ellie was described as being 'a very private person' who kept things to herself and found it difficult to make friends as she had very low self-confidence. She also had a very poor body image and throughout her admission, despite it being summer, wore thick, baggy clothes. It was believed that she had been verbally and possibly physically bullied at school.

Ellie was referred for individual music therapy because she was finding it difficult to express herself verbally and sometimes became confused by language. She also seemed to respond more positively in one-to-one situations than in a group. She had received music lessons in the past and played the piano, flute and clarinet.

Ellie came for weekly music therapy throughout her five months on the unit. During this time she discovered that she enjoyed improvising music with me and had a natural talent for it. Although she seemed very engaged, sometimes her music became quite repetitive and rhythmically rigid. She liked to 'get it [the music] right' and could become frustrated when she felt she was making mistakes. I wondered whether she needed *me* to create more structure around her playing to enable her to be more free. I introduced various structures to our music, such as the 12-bar blues and other harmonic progressions. She seemed to respond to this structured element and she was able to explore improvising in a more spontaneous way. I also encouraged her to think about whether our improvisations described anything or had a focus. She was able to suggest that we play in a certain key or style to reflect the mood she was in. I felt that this was important as Ellie generally talked so little about how she was feeling.

After a couple of months Ellie began to really develop a relationship with music and with me. She started bringing her clarinet and flute to the sessions, neither of which had she played for a long time. We played duets and she even showed me how to play the flute, which I did very badly! Perhaps it was helpful for Ellie to see me persevering with something unfamiliar and not worrying too much if I did not achieve immediate perfection. I wanted her to feel that she too could take risks and find a confidence to explore new ways of using music. Looking back on this case, what was happening during this early part of the therapy was that I was creating the 'right environment'. I feel that this was achieved through positive musical experiences, whereby Ellie felt heard and responded to, and also through the developing therapeutic relationship between us.

On one occasion Ellie arrived in tears. I asked her if she wanted to talk about anything. She replied 'No, I'm here for the music' and asked if we could 'just play'. We spent the entire session playing together. It seemed that the music room had become a place in which Ellie felt she could use music to express herself *with* someone else. She also started spending time on her own in the music room in the evenings. She told me that when she was feeling upset or angry, she liked to come and just play. Looking back on it, it was clear that she needed time to establish this relationship with music and to develop it in a variety of ways.

By this time Ellie had stopped attending the unit and was coming to music therapy as an outpatient. This change in her circumstances seemed to precipitate a change in direction for music therapy. We began to talk about music and about pop songs that were in the charts. I encouraged Ellie to think about why she liked them, and what it was about the music that interested her. It was also important that I knew something about the music that she was discussing so I suddenly found myself desperately trying to get into music ranging from Busted and Delta Goodrem to Evanescense and Eminem. We tried to recreate some of the music on various instruments but she was too self-conscious to sing. We also taped some of our improvisations, which she took home to listen to and play to her family. She was able to be quite analytical about the pieces and on one occasion said that she thought one of them would make a good song. I took this opportunity to suggest that we write a song together. She was keen and said she would start thinking about the lyrics. In this case, having encouraged Ellie's interest in songs, I then felt it was my role to facilitate her own writing of them. The therapy needed a new focus and songwriting seemed a natural progression.

We spent the next few weeks working on a song. The words came easily for Ellie and I was surprised by her imagination and clarity of thought. There is a strong feeling of melancholic longing in the lyrics, of time spent and wishes unheard. However, towards the end of the song she introduces an element of hope and manages to somehow 'save' her spirit and allow it to 'live again' (Figure 2.1).

At this point Ellie was more focused on the *lyrical* rather than the musical aspect of the process. The words flowed very easily for her and she wrote most of them in one session. As a result, my role was to help portray the ambience of the song through the music. I suggested a basic structure of verses and a chorus, and experimented on the piano with various motifs and phrases. I encouraged her to think and make decisions about the mood, style and other musical elements so that she would feel involved in the whole process. She wanted the song to sound melancholic up until the last chord so I suggested a minor key to create the right mood and a *tierce de Picardie* (final major chord) for a positive ending. We experimented with different keys, rhythmic patterns, dynamics and chords until arriving at what best suited the song. To my surprise, Ellie even tried out using her voice. Fortunately our voices were well matched in terms of range and timbre, which seemed to give her confidence.

We recorded the song at her request so that she could take it away with her. At this point I began to think about what function the song had in Ellie's life outside the sessions. Did it represent a part of her that she could not express in other situations? Did it represent something of which she was proud and was therefore a physical reminder that she was good at something?

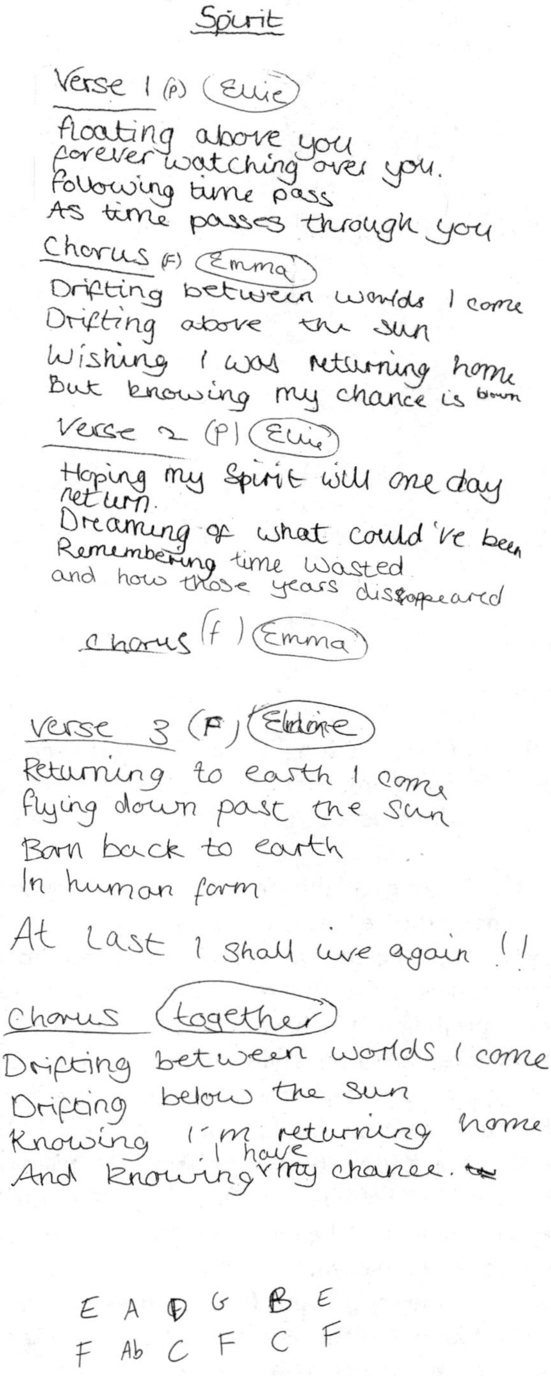

Spirit

Verse 1 (p) (Ellie)

floating above you
forever watching over you.
following time pass
As time passes through you

Chorus (f) (Emma)

Drifting between worlds I come
Drifting above the sun
Wishing I was returning home
But knowing my chance is gone

Verse 2 (p) (Ellie)

Hoping my spirit will one day
return.
Dreaming of what could've been
Remembering time wasted
and how those years disappeared

chorus (f) (Emma)

Verse 3 (F) (Eldone)

Returning to earth I come
Flying down past the sun
Born back to earth
In human form

At last I shall live again !!

Chorus (together)

Drifting between worlds I come
Drifting below the sun
Knowing I'm returning home
And knowing I have my chance.

E A D G B E
F Ab C F C F

Figure 2.1 'Spirit'

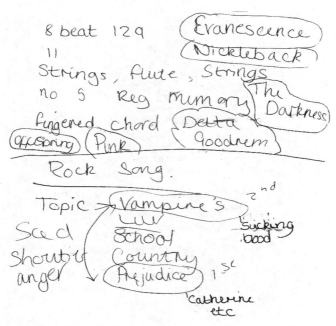

Figure 2.2 Brainstorming example

After the success of her first song 'Spirit', Ellie was keen to write another song. I encouraged her to brainstorm around some possible themes and she came up with vampires, love, school, asylum seekers/patriotism and prejudice (Figure 2.2).

We discussed each theme and the ideas and images they brought up for her. For example, the vampire theme led into a discussion about her fascination with blood and death which she decided would not make a good song. In the end she decided that she wanted us to focus on the theme of prejudice and write a song called 'The power of prejudice', which was one of three titles she had produced (Figure 2.3). When I asked her what style and mood she wanted, she said that she wanted it to be quite 'rocky and powerful'. I encouraged her to again think about some of the music to which she liked listening. She talked about a particular rock song she liked that had a repeated guitar riff. We tried out some riffs on a guitar but she did not feel it sounded 'rocky enough'. She commented that her father had an electric guitar that she might be able to borrow, which I thought was an excellent idea. The next week she arrived with the electric guitar and amplifier and we spent time trying out riffs and worked on creating the sound that she wanted. We found that the electric keyboard worked quite well with the electric guitar but the percussive instruments did not.

The process of trying things out but not always necessarily 'getting it right' was an important part of the process for Ellie. As previously mentioned, she

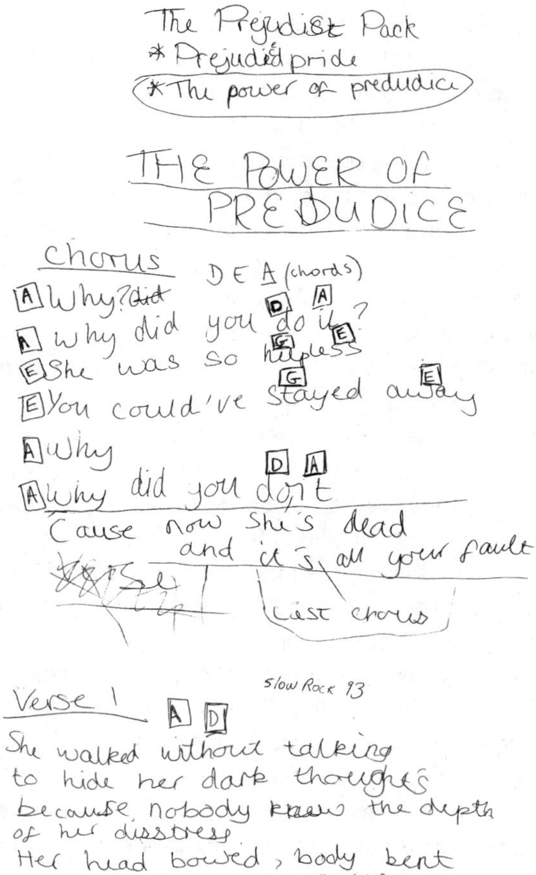

The Prejudist Pack
* Prejudist pride
(* The power of predudice)

THE POWER OF PREDUDICE

Chorus

D E A (chords)

[A] Why? did
[A] Why did you do it?
[E] She was so helpless
[E] You could've stayed away

[A] Why
[A] Why did you don't
'Cause now she's dead
and it's all your fault

~~* Sh~~

Last chorus

Slow Rock 93

Verse 1
[A] [D]

She walked without talking
to hide her dark thoughts
because nobody knew the depth
of her disstress.
Her head bowed, body bent
as if in constant prayer
And this is the story of a girl
called Claire.
Chorus

Verse 2

I went away and guess what,
found when I returned
She had slashed and slashed to
kill herself because of your
mental tortures the scars will
fade but never the power of prejudice

Chorus

Verse

Black is all you see at a funeral
And this is all I saw at Claire's
Because She slashed too deep
But you were the knife stole her
life

Figure 2.3 'The power of prejudice'

found it difficult to cope with things not being right. Now she was able to be more flexible and accept that things could not be perfect the first time around. Ellie also was able to contribute more actively to the musical side of the process. Perhaps in creating 'Spirit' she had gained confidence in her own abilities and was more willing to risk trying out ideas. Her lyrics for 'The power of prejudice' were extremely powerful and as she wrote them, I wondered whether she was actually describing something she had experienced at school and was using the girl in the song to represent herself (Figure 2.3).

Ellie performed her song at school, which gained her the attention of her music teacher and the respect of her peers. She started to use music therapy sessions to compose her own pieces with a little help from me. She was even asked to play one at her school leaving ceremony, which was something that she would have never done before. At her suggestion, she wanted the piece to 'describe' how she felt about leaving – a mixture of excitement and apprehension.

Creating her own music, whether songs or descriptive pieces, was starting to become an important part of Ellie's life and, as her mother commented, it was becoming 'Ellie's thing'. She even started to compose music at home and at school with peers. She received a lot of praise and encouragement from her family and school and appeared more self-confident. She even started to become more fashion conscious and developed an interest in clothes.

In this case, song-creating enabled Ellie to express some of the issues she was facing through a medium about which she felt confident. The clear structure of song appealed to her sense of order, yet the creative aspect gave her the opportunity to be flexible too. The fact that we were able to work together was an important part of the work as she usually found this difficult. The sessions worked with what Ellie was able to offer and, with my skills as a musician and therapist, we were able to create music of which we were both really proud. The process formed a transitional phase in the therapy before developing into other forms of composition. I feel that I have provided Ellie with a tool that she has mastered in her own way and will be able to carry on using in the future.

Case example: Matt's story

The following case describes how a young adolescent improvised his own songs during music therapy sessions with his mother. It demonstrates how flexible the form of song can be and how vital it was to create the right atmosphere to enable him to progress. The way my role developed, from a passive 'listening' role to a much more active musical role, will be discussed. The importance of recording and making the songs accessible beyond the therapy room is also highlighted.

Matt, a 13-year-old boy, was admitted to the Croft Unit for a six-week assessment of his severe behavioural and emotional difficulties. The high level of violence and aggression he displayed, particularly towards his mother, was becoming a great cause for concern as were his extreme low moods. He was finding it very difficult to cope at school and was attending only on a part-time basis. His behaviour seemed to have deteriorated since several bereavements and crises within his family. He found it very difficult to talk about his problems and would often become muddled and frustrated when trying to explain what was wrong. He had been slow to develop speech as a child and still had moments of poor articulation.

During the admission it became clear that Matt had a very complex relationship with his mother. When she was not at the unit, he would become very upset and worry that something bad would happen to her. However, when she did come, he would become very rude and aggressive towards her. They had very few positive times together and Matt's mum was finding it increasingly difficult to manage his difficult behaviour.

Matt began to show an interest in music during the weekly music therapy group. Despite his extremely low self-esteem he was nevertheless able to let himself engage with and enjoy music-making, both on his own and with others. On one occasion, following an angry outburst at one of the nurses, he wrote her a poem entitled 'How I feel' which he brought to the group (Figure 2.4). He wanted to perform it to her whilst accompanying himself on the guitar.

I began to reflect on why he was able to *sing* an apology and explain how he felt but not able to verbalize it.

I began to see Matt and his mother together for music therapy sessions. The multidisciplinary team were interested in how they interacted together through a non-verbal medium as they seemed to find it very difficult to communicate with each other in conventional ways. I also wondered whether Matt would be able to use his aptitude for poem- or songwriting to express some of his feelings to his mother.

During our first session together Matt spontaneously sang to both his mother and me. He sang of his happiness that he was in the music room and of what he would like to do. I was surprised that he was confident enough to sing in front of us both as he was usually very self-conscious. As the session progressed Matt and his mother were able to have some positive interactions within the music and even giggled together as we took it in turns to 'catch' each other out during a musical game. It seemed that the music was able to engage them on a different level than other interventions and enable them to play with one another.

Over the next few weeks singing began to form an integral part of the sessions. During the opening greeting song, Matt sang about his time on the unit and I responded by singing questions or responses to him. He was able to tell us

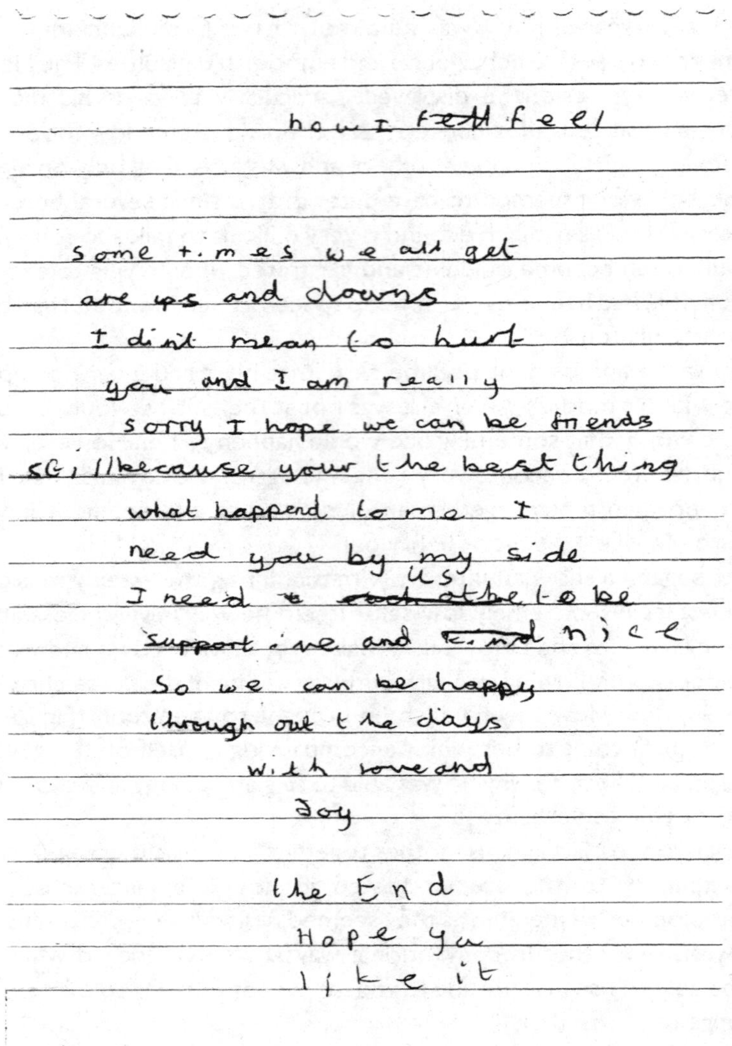

how I ~~fell~~ feel

some times we all get
are ups and downs
I din't mean to hurt
you and I am really
sorry I hope we can be friends
so, ~~I~~ because your the best thing
what happend to me   I
need you by my side
                          us
I need ~~to~~ ~~coth atbe~~ to be
support·ive and ~~k·nd~~ nice
So we can be happy
through out the days
with love and
Joy

the End
Hope ya
like it

Figure 2.4 'How I feel'

some of the difficulties he was facing as well as some of the things he was enjoying. Singing appeared to be something with which he felt at ease and which came quite naturally to him.

Due to his extremely low self-esteem and inability to regulate his emotions, Matt found it very difficult to cope with things that went wrong. He would become very upset at school if, for example, he made a mistake in his writing or a piece of artwork and could not accept encouragement to move on. What surprised me in music therapy sessions was that Matt found it easier to accept what he perceived as 'mistakes' in his playing. Although he needed some verbal encouragement from me at times, he seemed to be able to try things out in the music that did not always work the first time. I have often found that children are able to risk ideas and tolerate making mistakes in music more than in other settings. Perhaps it is due to the fact that the mistakes are not visible, like they may be in a piece of writing or artwork, and are therefore less threatening.

Over the next few weeks Matt tried out many different instruments and ways of playing. I worked hard at reflecting his musical ideas within my playing to give him an experience of being heard and valued. Sometimes when he became frustrated and on the verge of giving up, saying that his music was 'rubbish' and mine was 'better', I told him that it was *his* music that was enabling me to play and giving me ideas. He responded positively to this and we were able to continue.

What was important throughout this time was that Matt felt he could trust me, the situation and the music. He needed to know that we could tolerate whatever he needed to express – even if that meant playing extremely loudly and drowning out our playing completely. He needed to know that I would listen and still be there for him the next week. It also felt important that Matt's mother was there to listen to him too. I wanted Matt to feel that we could both hear and accept his way of expressing himself.

Matt missed the last few days of his admission because of illness. However, he returned with his mother to the unit for a farewell party and a music therapy session. They arrived late which Matt was very agitated about. He blamed his mother and hit out at her, becoming quite violent. Eventually he calmed down enough to get himself to the music room but he continued to look very agitated and on the verge of losing control. I felt that there was nothing I could say that could help the situation so I simply picked up two guitars, handed one to him and began to strum quietly. Matt joined in and we played together for some time until he looked visibly calmer. He told us that he would like to sing a song and asked whether we would just sit and listen. Matt had no words written down, he just sang as his feelings and ideas came to him, accompanying himself on the guitar. His song was in a rap style. What follows are the words I later transcribed.

I hate to break it to you,
not everyone's perfect.
If they were, they weren't normal.
Sometimes people have their ups and downs
Sometimes...even, sometimes they have their bad times
because I'll tell you.

Once the worst thing in my life was...

It was a normal day
I was round my Auntie's
We were watching TV
and my mum got a phone call.
It was someone saying that my Nan was in an accident
And they said, 'Sorry to say this, but she has passed away.'
And people say that at least she's in a good place
and that she has peace and quiet.

We all missed her
We froze like a bomb had just dropped on our house
And that was the worst day of my life.

And then I thought, what was the worst thing
What's the other worse things that are going to happen to me?

But then after a couple of months,
I began to get over it.
People said, 'Just cheer up and put your head up high
and say that's it's not the end of the world.'

But I feel that it is

Then my Auntie got rushed into hospital
because she had some cancer
Then that was the next worst thing that happened to me, my mum and my
family.
But luckily, just by a…(?)
she recovered.
She put up a fight.
I bet she said to herself,
'I'm not going to give up.
I've got people who care about me.
I'm not going to give up.'

So when she came out of hospital
it was like a miracle,
I said a *miracle*.
Before I didn't believe in miracles
but when they started to happen,
I said to myself, 'Thank you, God.'

But then just as things were looking up,
she had it again.
And I was fed up.

I was just sitting in my room just thinking,
'What other stuff can happen in my life?'

But then she had her operation
to make herself better
and it worked.
And then she came out of the hospital again.
She looked like a new woman
and my mum was so glad.
She didn't need this tragedy again,
she didn't need this, this sad thing to happen again.

But sometimes me and my Auntie have arguments
and I say some horrible stuff.
But she knows that I don't mean it
and I regret it when I say some horrible stuff
because I know that she wouldn't…(?)…

But then after that I was getting on fine.
I thought that the worst days were gone.
Then I saw the sun shining, comes out after…(?)…

It's like we're trapped in a [tank?]
with loads of the worst things that could happen.

My sister had an accident.
I was playing out with friends
and when I came in for a drink,
the door was locked.
No one was home.

So I went to Tina's (that's Grace's house).
I said, 'Where's my mum and where's my sister?'
She said, 'They're at the hospital. I'm sorry to say that your sister is in hospital,
she tried to commit suicide.'

And then again I froze.
Like someone's just…froze me and dumped me in a giant freezer.
I was as stiff as a stick.

Then my mum phoned up and I was crying to her.
And I said, 'Why? Why did she do it?'
But my mum don't know why
and she still don't know why
because Christina don't tell us,
cos she don't think she can.

I can't do anything.

And if I find out that someone has done anything to her.
Then I said to her, 'Why can't you tell us?
It'll make you better.'
And I said, 'If I get my hands on the person who done something to you,
they will regret it to their graves.'

And when she came out of hospital
after a couple of weeks,
she looked like nothing can happen.

So, there you go,
another miracle has happened
and I hold my head up high and I say, 'Thank you, God.'

So I'm singing this song so you don't get your hopes up
and say that I've got a perfect life, but…
Don't count on it because something bad might happen,
like my family.
And I don't forget these miracles that he gave me.

The atmosphere after he sang was a stunned silence emanating from Matt's mother and myself. Matt had not talked about these issues that were worrying him and suddenly, on his last day, after a difficult journey to the unit, he was communicating things that had been worrying him for such a long time. Matt's mother clearly found it difficult to know what to say which Matt immediately took as her not liking his song. She had to reassure him that this was not the case, just that it was difficult for her to hear how upset he was. Matt then asked whether he could sing his song again, only this time he wanted me to tape it. He was then able to take the tape away with him. It felt important that Matt had his song to keep and could decide what he wanted to do with it.

  After the session I felt quite overcome but also amazed that Matt has been able to use the medium of a song to express his fears and feelings whereas he had been unable to talk about them. What was it about singing that enabled him to do this? Was it the fact that singing felt less threatening to him and less likely to end in frustration than talking? Generally the words of a song come slower than when talking, so for someone who has difficulties talking, the time and space that the act of singing provides can be easier to work with. Certainly I found this the case when I worked with a stroke victim who could hardly string a sentence together but could sing verses of songs perfectly. In Matt's case it seemed that by creating something out of his anxieties that could be heard by others, he was putting them in a more manageable form.

Through the expansion of the music therapy provision at the unit, I was able to offer Matt and his mother sessions on an outpatient basis to start two months later. They have now been coming for eight months. Matt continues to be able to use song as a way to express himself, even when he is extremely upset about something. On one occasion they arrived very late because the taxi driver had to pick up someone else and had got lost. Matt chose instruments that he told us represented different parts of the driver's body. He sang about his anger towards the man and used the instruments to 'hit' him. Although it was a very violent song and hard to listen to, especially for Matt's mother, it was a more constructive way of expressing himself than by physically hitting out, which he was inclined to do.

As the sessions have progressed Matt has begun to express many of his difficulties through his improvised songs. He has sung songs about his relationships with peers at school and how hurt he feels, for example, when friendships break up. He has also sung about the more positive times he experiences; for example, he improvised a song called 'The happy song' which he sang for his mother. At my suggestion he has also engaged in improvised story-telling where he 'sings' a story which we both accompany with piano and percussive music. During one story, after a long, complicated battle, he emerged as 'Matt the Great', the 'rescuer' who saved the other characters in his story. It is through these different song forms that we have been able to gain an insight into the way Matt relates to people and to his environment and therefore find ways in which to help him.

The most useful thing that music therapy is able to offer in this case is a safe space in which Matt can express whatever he feels without any pressure. In a way I have merely facilitated this space and made sure that both Matt and his mother know that I can listen and accept what Matt brings. I have also, I hope, made Matt realize that he has a real talent for expressing himself through song which could have a positive knock-on effect and go some way to increasing his self-confidence. For Matt's mother, too, it has been a very positive experience to be able to observe him doing something creative that he enjoys. She often talks about the fact that they can barely be in the same room with one another without a fight or argument occurring, yet in music therapy they seem to be able to communicate and even enjoy being together.

Evaluating the process

As part of the song-creating process, I encourage each child to complete a short questionnaire about their experiences (Figure 2.5). Questions such as why song-writing is enjoyable, whether it can be useful and whether it continues to play a part in their lives outside the sessions are addressed. The aim of this questionnaire is to inform me, in the children's own words, how they felt about the whole process. Both

Ellie and Matt highlighted the fact that they were able to express themselves through their songs. Matt commented, '[Songwriting] helps me share some of my feelings. It's relaxing and if I'm in a mood, it calms me down.' Ellie commented that she enjoyed songwriting because she 'could tell emotions/thoughts' and she thought it was useful as it gave her 'something to think about'. Both identified that they continued to write songs outside the music therapy sessions. Matt told me that he had been 'rapping' his own songs at home but the words were 'a bit rude' so he thought he better not sing them to me!

I find the questionnaire a very valuable source of information as, although it is clear to *me* that songwriting can form an important and useful part of music therapy, it is really helpful to hear the child's perspective.

Concluding thoughts

In this chapter I have explored the valuable role that song-creating can play for children with complex emotional and behavioural difficulties. For many of my clients it can be one of the few ways in which they are able to express themselves and share some of the difficulties which they are facing. Many have very low self-esteem and feel that they are unable to achieve anything positive. Through the creative process of song-creating they find that they *can* achieve something and many discover that they actually have a natural talent. This can clearly be an extremely rewarding experience for both the children and their families.

In each case a song creation makes a different journey. Some start and finish in the music room, some travel with the child to their homes or schools. Some are used as an interface between themselves and others when they are not yet ready to communicate verbally. In every case I feel my role is to facilitate and encourage a process that the children can use not only in music therapy but in their lives outside.

I would like to find out what you thought about writing songs whilst at the Croft. By telling me what you think, you can help other people understand how useful writing songs can be.

1.   Had you ever written a song before coming to music therapy?   Yes ☐   No ☐

2.   Did you enjoy writing songs?   Yes ☐   No ☐

     What was the reason?

3.   Did you find writing songs useful?   Yes ☐   No ☐

     Why was this?

4.   What did you find easier?
     Writing the words ☐   Writing the music? ☐

5.   Was there anything that helped you think of words for   Yes ☐   No ☐
     your song?

6.   Was there anything that helped you with the music for   Yes ☐   No ☐
     the song?

7.   Was there a band/singer/song that helped you write   Yes ☐   No ☐
     your song?
     If so, please write which ones.

8.   Have you written any songs when you are not in music   Yes ☐   No ☐
     therapy?

     If yes, can you say what your song was about?

Thank you very much for answering these questions.

Figure 2.5 Songwriting feedback questionnaire

3

Teenagers and Songwriting

Supporting Students
in a Mainstream Secondary School

Philippa Derrington

Songwriting can be a useful way to help teenagers put ideas together cohesively and creatively. All teenagers relate to music at some level and respond well to the structure which songs provide. This chapter will look at how teenagers' rhetoric and emotions can be expressed and channelled in songs, why songwriting is an important intervention, and what happens in sessions to help this process come about. Different ways in which the therapist facilitates students' work is then illustrated in four short case examples.

Music therapy in a mainstream secondary school

I work as a music therapist at Cottenham Village College, which is a mainstream secondary school in Cambridgeshire, UK, with 1000 students aged between 11 and 16. It has a large Student Support Centre supporting students with special developmental, emotional and behavioural needs. The aim of the Centre is to provide alternative lessons for students, often on a one-to-one basis, to equip them socially as well as academically for reintegration into mainstream classes. Students at particular risk include those who are in care, who live in families under stress, who are frequently suspended from school, travellers and young carers. Music therapy has become an established service within the school providing either a short-term or long-term provision for students, the majority of whom attend the Centre. However, other students who only attend the main school can be referred for music therapy if there is concern for their emotional state.

Identifying students' needs

Students are referred to music therapy for various reasons, but primarily to offer additional emotional support and assistance in identifying difficulties which they are experiencing. Aims of therapy depend on each student's needs but, typically, may be to decrease tension, anxiety or challenging behaviour, provide students with insight into the meaning of their behaviour, and provide an effective means for self-expression. While group work would be beneficial, I work with students on a one-to-one basis due to the limitations of the size of the room and I find that students respond positively to time out from the busy environment and peer pressure, to a space where they choose what to do, how to work and can set their own pace.

As teenage students develop their own identity and sense of self, conflict can arise between the individual's needs and societal expectations. Eriksson's statement that 'developing youths…are now primarily concerned with what they appear to be in the eyes of others as compared with what they feel they are' (1963, p.253) can be constantly observed in the school environment. However, the therapeutic space enables teenagers to express themselves and try out new ways of communicating and relating to another person in a safe and confidential way.

Using songs and songwriting helps affirm this exploration of self and how it relates to others. Most of the time teenagers are engaged in socially related activities and see all they do as a social role. If their definition of self is through a social role, as Eriksson (1968) suggests, then it explains why songwriting is effective because songs are often produced with listeners in mind. For example, songs may be created for a particular person, notably a member of teaching or support staff, and it is interesting that students who are often in conflict with certain teachers want to write songs specifically for them. Songwriting is a social activity as it is a shared process between student and therapist, even if the therapist is actively listening rather than playing or singing, and students learn to feel accepted for who they are and to know that their expression is heard and acknowledged.

Theoretical framework

Students are encouraged to experiment with the instruments and to express themselves through the use of sound in whichever way they choose, such as listening to music, playing on their own or improvising together. Following the Alvin model of free improvisation (Wigram *et al.* 2002, p.130) I usually do not impose guidelines to an improvisation but allow the student to design it. Occasionally, depending on the student, it is necessary to be more directive and lead specific musical activities or ideas; however, for most students the free improvisational model works well in supporting every aspect of self-expression that they bring to a session.

> Alvin sought to establish *equal term* relationships with her clients. In an equal term relationship, the therapist and client share musical experiences at the same level and have equal control over the musical situation. (Bruscia 1987, p.77)

Although I work in a student-centred way, I follow Alvin's principle that the musical relationship is a combined effort and that all music counts. Alvin also put emphasis on creating a positive mood in the present which is an essential way to work with teenagers. It is really important that teenagers enjoy their sessions because they would simply stop attending if they were not motivated. Once they trust and accept the therapist and setting, teenagers can be very enthusiastic about the project of writing a song which contradicts the apathy so often accredited to them.

The function and value of songwriting with teenagers

Songs versus free improvisation

Even though students are introduced to the music therapy setting as a space and time to improvise and use instruments experimentally, all students enjoy using songs in some way and many students create songs of their own on a regular basis. The concept of free improvisation may seem alien and exposing to the teenager who has rarely, or never, experimented with instruments, and who feels inhibited by a student-centred approach to working. Students are used to the routine of a mainstream secondary school, organized by rules and timetables, which can explain why they often turn to the structure of songs and the project of songwriting. Whereas free improvisation can feel unpredictable and odd, teenagers, who are used to discipline and structure, can find songwriting purposeful and satisfying.

Songs are a means of using everyday language imaginatively

 Teenagers in a mainstream environment are used to articulate and verbal forms of communication, so it seems a natural progression that they should want to add words to music to communicate how they see themselves and what they are feeling. Words are distinct and can be explicit in defining music (Storr 1992), which should suggest that songwriting would be more exposing than free improvisation, yet words are the teenagers' primary means of communication. 'Teenagers are still forming an identity and learning that the words they have learnt or choose to use are an element of their character and identity' (Round 2001, p.15). Thus, communicating through song lyrics, using their everyday language, is a reliable way for teenagers to express themselves. Words in the form of lyrics can be easier and less confrontational to handle than conversation, especially if they are thinking about, and wanting to share, difficult issues. It can also be noted that the effect of writing lyrics can alter students' instinctive tendency to use bad language and inspire them to think of other words and images.

Songs express opinion, emotions and develop ideas

Songwriting increases students' confidence and independence. The production of a song can provide a real sense of achievement. It can help turn around negative ways of relating to others into positive interactions because the work is a shared process and based on the therapeutic paradigm of listening and supporting. The subject matter in songs can be negative and sometimes violent but the structured and interactive work of putting ideas into song is a therapeutic intervention, which is managed in the confidential and containable therapy setting.

It is interesting how frequently nursery rhymes or other children's songs are incorporated into teenagers' music and song creation. When the therapeutic environment feels safe enough to do this, teenagers can re-run playful ideas regardless of not being age appropriate and can use songs to meet their emotional need without being affected by peer pressure.

Introducing songs

The content of students' sessions varies a great deal depending on the influences that they bring and how they want to use their time. This is why there are different ways of capturing the teenagers' imagination with the idea of songwriting. I usually introduce the idea in the first couple of sessions and anticipate that students will return to the idea when they want to. Most students want to use songs and will look at song books which are in the room, but they do not always consider the possibility of songwriting.

The stages of songwriting

Once students decide to write a song, which I describe as stage 1, they follow one of two routes. These approaches are outlined next:

First approach

Stage 1 Decision to write a song

Stage 2 Talk about themes, ideas and intentions

Stage 3 Draw on different sources for lyrics

> For example:
>
> > (a) use pre-composed lyrics
> >
> > (b) use play
> >
> > (c) use prepared material

Stage 4 Write down lyrics

Stage 5 Talk about ideas and effects for music composition

> For example:
>
> > (a) use pre-composed melodies
> >
> > (b) use familiar chord sequences

Stage 6 Write down score

Stage 7 Make a recording and update song folder

This first approach helps students think systematically about the song they want to create; however, not every stage is used, nor are they necessarily in this order. Instead, students are encouraged to consider each stage but construct songs in their own way. By directing students to immediately focus on the lyrics first, they are less likely to move away from the idea and get distracted by jamming. Therefore students are encouraged to talk about issues and themes they want to put in the song (stage 2) and to concentrate on one or two of them. Themes which students suggest often focus on the present and are therefore to do with everyday life such as how they are feeling about school, how they manage relationships with others at home, with friends and how they see themselves. It can be useful to discuss a student's intentions for writing a song and whether they have a specific audience in mind, and whether they are hoping to share it with anyone when it is completed.

Stage 3 begins to look at the different sources which inspire students to write lyrics. Their inspiration may be drawn from pre-composed lyrics (3a), and students are encouraged to share lyrics from songs to which they relate in a particular way. Lyrics from pop songs, for example, can be a valuable and easily accessible source for teenagers to use as a way of representing themselves and communicating their feelings. They can also serve as a model which students can adapt without having to start their own lyrics from scratch.

Songs can also be inspired by play (3b). Engaging in role-play and acting out can be the starting block for a song and an imaginative way of creating lyrics. Besides musical instruments, other equipment in the music therapy room can be used for play, such as puppets, pretend mobile phones, art materials and a classroom whiteboard.

Due to the school environment where students are used to homework and consider it normal to prepare written material, it is not uncommon for students to arrive with lyrics which they have prepared ahead of their music therapy session or written within another class (such as poetry written for an English class, 3c). Whatever sources students bring with them, such as CDs, games or prepared lyrics, it shows that students will take responsibility for the content of their sessions and that they anticipate and are engaged in the songwriting process.

As students gather their thoughts together for lyrics, I listen and respond empathically. Talking about the theme and reflecting back ideas for lyrics can help to keep their focus. I also offer ways of formatting the ideas, for example, by creating phrasing, rhyming lines, separating verses, creating a chorus or a coda. Although the process of composing a song is a shared one, the inspiration for lyrics is theirs and I try to help them shape their work without imposing on their self-expression. On a practical level, I make sure that lyrics are written down or recorded (stage 4) and this may involve typing up lyrics in time for the following session, as well as keeping individual song folders up to date, for students to look back on and refer to.

Once the lyrics are formed, students are encouraged to think about the musical composition, described as stage 5. Many students play instruments, such as the guitar or small percussion instruments, while they are writing lyrics and may already have an idea of the musical effects that they want to create. However, they often need more assistance to think about melody, rhythm and dynamics and I encourage them to do this by experimenting on different instruments and talking about how they want the song to be musically constructed.

Students draw on different sources to create music. For example, the melody could be taken from a pre-composed song, or even from a ring tone on a mobile phone. Listening to pre-recorded music which they bring to a session can be a good starting point for adapting or recreating songs as well as generating conversation and discussion about their musical taste and favourite bands. This is important to know before assisting with any musical composition. Teenagers are inventive and introduce new ideas all the time, which is why it is appropriate to have a flexible approach of incorporating both pre-composed and improvised music in song-writing as a way of embracing teenagers' resources.

Following all the leads that I am given for the style, melody, pitch, rhythm and dynamics, I experiment and improvise with a musical composition. Students will normally correct me if it does not sound right or accurately reflect their own intentions. The musical key is determined by the student's vocal range and if they want to create a melody that they can sing or play while I support them on the clarinet or improvise around their tune with simple chord sequences on the piano. Rhythm is very important and a strong beat can be a good way of trimming lyrics into a structured and succinct format.

Some students want to play and include ideas with which they are familiar from school music lessons. Simple chord sequences such as I–IV–V–I, which they have learnt on the piano, can become the base for the musical composition. This pattern of moving from the tonic to the subdominant, to the dominant (or dominant seventh) and returning to the tonic, can be exemplified in the key of C major as C–F–G–C. Similarly, familiar patterns such as Boogie-Woogie (with a chord sequence of I–IV–I–V–IV–I which, in the key of C major, is C–F–C–G–F–C) are popular with students.

Writing down the musical score is the next stage (stage 6) in the songwriting process which can be done on manuscript paper or the white board. Students who can read music or know letter names of notes can write up a score of the basic chord pattern or melody, whereas others may use diagrams. For example, one student drew lots of recorder finger charts on the board to remember a melody that she had created and from which she could read.

Having created the lyrics and music, students decide and direct how the song is to be played. This may be played through several times, indeed over several sessions, but the aim is often to create a recording and a final version (stage 7). Students can use the recording equipment, which includes minidisc and a video camera, and therefore decide and control what to record. For some, it is important to record material at earlier stages of songwriting because listening back to their songs together can help students to reflect on their feelings and help to clarify and validate them.

As well as using students' own song folders for this purpose, listening back to recordings is another way that reminds students of what they were doing in previous sessions and allows a song, which has been started, to be re-addressed, added to and possibly changed. Some songs may be aborted or have a sudden ending because ideas can change and they may dislike work they have previously done. Even though some recordings may be destroyed, the on-going process of making recordings does help to substantiate the process of songwriting and provide palpable evidence of their work.

Second approach

Students often follow another approach to songwriting and that is to improvise the whole process first before looking at the song in more detail, as outlined below.

Stage 1 Decision to write a song

Stage 2 Create music and lyrics simultaneously in improvised and free-flowing forms of expression

Stage 3 Talk about song

The here and now is very important to teenagers and songwriting can be fast, spontaneous and an active way to express themselves. The nature of an improvised song can tap into emotions in an immediate way and their words, which may not be premeditated, can express a thought, feeling or be the result of a recent situation. Students might play an instrument to act as a supportive background while I accompany these songs on a different instrument and may reflect back their lyrics by singing. After an improvised song I encourage the student to talk about the song, its meaning and intention, and I will suggest that it can be transcribed or recorded.

However, if students decide to put together the musical score and effects, I consider myself to be co-musician who follows their lead, listens, responds musically and talks with them about the overall composition. Teenagers' moods and thoughts can sometimes change very quickly and drastically but, by listening to them and being aware of the styles of music which they enjoy, supporting their lyrics with improvised music can keep up with, and track these moods, responding quickly in style, dynamics and tempi.

Case examples

The following case examples illustrate different ways in which students create songs but follow this therapeutic paradigm of encouraging, listening, sharing and supporting.

Case example: 'Somewhere over the rainbow'

To illustrate the way in which pre-composed songs can be used, I will describe the work with a 15-year-old student who has mild learning difficulties and attends both mainstream classes and the Student Support Centre for lessons. I introduced the idea of songwriting to her in the third session and she seemed hesitant of the idea. The following week she arrived with tapes of soundtracks to musicals, and set about singing along to them. The lyrics of the songs she chose were all about having ambition and being in love, and she seemed reassured by the familiarity of each song's length, melody and lyrics which she knew by heart.

Recreating the songs seemed a very important way for her to express how she was feeling and gave her a sense of achievement. She did not play any instruments but sang with a microphone and pretended to be on a television talent games show. She introduced her performance as now 'live on stage' which was the only time during the session that she communicated directly with me. This pattern of behaviour was repeated for several sessions and it was clearly a positive experience, to which she looked forward.

She gradually began to talk to me about other things that concerned her, as well as continuing with performances and announcing the songs she was going to sing. I used this opportunity to suggest that she could add her own lyrics to these songs and include some of the things she had been talking about. She flatly refused such an idea but returned the following week and changed some of the lyrics as she sang, introducing her own words to the melody and structure of these songs.

Somewhere over the rainbow
There is a handsome boy
Coming to win his heart
To fall in love with me

I have a new rainbow
Filled with special colours
I wish for a heart
I wish for my golden rainbow.

Lyrics inspired by pre-composed song 'Somewhere Over the Rainbow'
from The Wizard of Oz (L. Frank Baum, 1903)

Rather than verbalize another suggestion, I decided to play one of the songs on the piano at the start of the next session. In this way I was able to engage her with live music but which was familiar to her and distracted her from playing tapes straight away. From this point, her songs began to take on an independent form of expression but with a recognizable style as she sang and I accompanied her. Initially I played the songs as they were written but gradually introduced more improvisation and which allowed her to create lyrics that did not scan with the original melody but could move away to create her own song. Having been inspired by her favourite genre of music, the student could adapt songs and interweave her own words with the official lyrics. Figure 3.1 is the first verse that she wrote and sang to a tune which was accompanied on the piano with sequences of predictable broken chords. She wrote down the lyrics and liked the idea of beginning a song folder but she also recorded the song onto tape which she could take away with her and play to others.

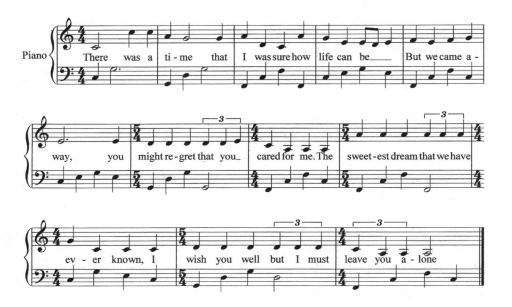

Figure 3.1 'There was a time'

Case example: 'Love song'

When I began work with 14-year-old Sally, I introduced the idea of songwriting to her and she responded enthusiastically. She had lots of ideas which I listened to and discussed with her, before helping her to concentrate on one theme in particular. She decided that the first song she would write would be a love song for her boyfriend and she talked to me about how she felt about doing this. Initially Sally seemed overwhelmed by ideas for the lyrics that she wanted to include so I took one or two lines and suggested shorter phrases for each of them, which she immediately started to experiment with by singing. As she did this, I added a quiet piano accompaniment and played chords to support the phrasing. I chose the key of F major to which she seemed to relate easily. She continued in this way, trying out other lines of lyrics and repeating them in shorter phrases until she was happy with each one. I sang some lines back to her which she could reflect on, accept or reject. Once or twice our singing overlapped and this seemed to encourage Sally as her singing became stronger, more confident and sure of the melody which she was creating. This process took two sessions of 45 minutes, and at the end the lyrics were written down.

Love song

Baby you're the only one
I have never felt this way before
When you are around I feel all cold
And I can't be myself.
If you wanna be with me
You have got to prove it
And it's all I want is for everything to be alright.

Cos all I need is your love
And your trust
Baby we could sort this out
And make a new start
Cos all I wanna do is be with you
When I'm around you I feel safe
Cos I know you'll protect me.
Baby I love you
And I don't want anyone else but you.

Listening to Sally's singing suggested that she wanted to create a pop love song. She always began with the same note but asked for me to give her an introductory chord. I accompanied her song in a ballad style which I felt would match her singing and then we discussed it before the final piano part was decided upon. This accompaniment was then recorded because Sally wanted us to include other instruments in the composition. Sally tried various versions of the song and experimented with sounds and effects using different instruments. Each version was recorded on minidisc so that we could listen back and discuss the result. One version was more rhythmic and included the drum kit and castanets; however, she decided that the final version should be sung with accompanying piano, guitar and egg shakers.

Case example: From play to song

The following is an example of a song written which emerged as a result of play. The 15-year-old student used finger puppets and an improvised stage, which was set up with a table and sheet. He chatted about how he was going to create the song but not about the content of the lyrics. Once we had set up the stage together and arranged which instrument I would play, he began. He sang in the first person but could distance himself from the story and its lead character by telling it symbolically through song and by working underneath the table and therefore be out of sight.

He arranged his stage so he could see me when he needed to and used hand signals to tell me exactly when to start and stop the musical accompaniment on the keyboard. I followed his directions, his singing and the puppets' movements with simple chords in the Phrygian mode, moving between E minor and F major. He set up the video very carefully to record the show, but did not want anything to be written down or for this song to be included in his song folder. Enthusiasm for his activity and my equal involvement in the song with music validated his demonstrative play.

I am the robber
I am the robber, I am the robber
Robbing, riding round the city
I am the robber, getting all the jewellery.
What is here, behind my back?
But what, what, what is that?
I don't know, do you?
I am a thief who steals
Anything except for…
The only thing that I catch is
Money, jewels and credit cards
And stop!
And then I…thieve jewels
I thieve, I am a thief
You are not a thief
Say goodbye jewellery […]

I am not afraid of anyone, anyone, anyone, anyone, anyone, anyone, anyone
Except for cats, cats, cats, cats
Miaow, miaow
What was that?…
Cats!…AARGHH!

Case example: From school work to song

Songs enable teenagers to play with new ideas and schemes, without necessarily having to identify with any one in particular. The next excerpt is taken from a song entitled 'Perry the skunk', which was created by a student who had just come from a biology lesson where he had learned about animal testing. On arrival in the music therapy room, he told me about his opinion on animal testing and began to sing a song. He launched straight into an improvised song and, strumming the guitar, sang using Sprechgesang. By gesture he directed me to join in with the drums as he sang it through a second time and I added a beat which supported his lyrics. He was pleased with the effect and set about making an audio recording so that he could share it with a friend. He also wrote the lyrics down afterwards. This is an example of how the second approach to songwriting is an effective way for students to express themselves spontaneously and to provide an opportunity to talk about it afterwards.

Hey, Mr Science Guy

Hey, Mr Science Guy
Don't spray that aerosol in my eye
I don't really want to die
Get that rabbit away from the cage
I am filled with a lot of rage
I know you're only doing it for a decent wage

Lyrics by Jamie

Considerations and recommendations for work with teenagers

Choice, control and containment

How should the therapist play and to what extent? Teenagers appreciate being in charge and soon recognize that music therapy sessions are student-centred which is often in direct contrast to other educational aspects of school life. Consequently, they can be quick to criticize and refute any suggestions made by the therapist. Sometimes it can be very difficult to gauge how much input to give to students and how much to leave to their experimentation, but enthusiasm and encouragement is always recommended! Adolescent students essentially require choice, control and containment (De Backer 1993; Flower 1993) and they usually know exactly how they want things to be. They become quickly frustrated if the song does not 'sound right'.

It can be difficult to follow their instruction or interpret this correctly, which can raise issues of control similar to those which students experience in other settings. As Oldfield (1993) describes in her work with families, issues of control with different family members can be dealt with in musical activities. In the same way, creating songs with teenagers about school or their family can address difficult issues such as tension between siblings, conflict with teaching staff or bullying. Students have the opportunity to be in control and be the director and learn to express their intentions and ideas in a structured and succinct way.

Structure and purpose

Teenagers benefit from the process of songwriting because it is an effective way for them to express and define themselves in a format which meets their emotional needs in an organized and productive way. Whilst students recognize that they determine the choice and direction which their song takes, they also need to feel that the process is an organized one. Without some order of time and clear purpose the experience can evoke anxiety and may be rubbished, because it feels unusual and the therapist is considered a freak (McFerran 2003).

The intended purpose for many students' songs is for them to be heard by others. I am sometimes assigned to be a family member or teacher who must listen to the song, or may be a member of their band, who must follow their leadership exactly. In a more direct way, some students play or sing noticeably louder when they see somebody walking past the room. Music filters across to other school buildings, even if the windows are shut because 'music's sound and energy naturally leaks out from its source' (Pavlicevic and Ansdell 2004, p.16). Some students let others hear their recordings and others are keen to take part in school concerts. Carrying their work over to the main school is a useful way to support and include students in mainstream activities.

Conclusion

As in the case with improvisation, all songs function as a means of self-expression. The added element of performance and the possibility of sharing recordings is important to teenagers who put so much emphasis on social status and others' opinions. Songwriting is a way of creating music in a structured and coherent way, which is meaningful and helpful to teenagers in the mainstream setting as they discover new ways of defining their thoughts, developing ideas in creative ways and learning to recognize that their expression has value and meaning, which needs to be acknowledged by themselves as well as others.

4

Giving a Voice to Childhood Trauma through Therapeutic Songwriting

Toni Day

This chapter provides an overview of the therapeutic songwriting technique used with individuals who have experienced childhood abuse, in externalizing painful stories from their past along with creating a greater awareness for clients of the impact of childhood abuse on their current lives. It has developed through work completed by the author and her social work colleague, over a period of several years, with women who have experienced all forms of physical, sexual and psychological violence throughout their childhoods and into their adult lives. It begins by discussing the rationale for using group songwriting methods with adult survivors of child abuse, the multi-disciplinary nature of the work, and continues to describe the process of song creation through to recording and the performance of their work. A case example will be utilized to highlight important aspects of song creation with this client population, many of whom have spent most of their lives struggling to find their voices after enduring a lifetime of silence and secrecy.

Childhood abuse and its impact

Child abuse constitutes a form of stress that holds an inordinately high potential to have a traumatizing impact upon both the child victim in its immediate aftermath and the adult survivor across the life span (Courtois 1988). Instead of being nurtured as children, adult survivors of childhood abuse have often lived being subjected to daily routines of control and rejection. They may experience feelings such as fear, shock, disbelief or a doubting of their own memories or reactions. They may suffer from a sense of powerlessness, shame and embarrassment, and may fear that no-one would believe them or want to know. They can also feel bouts of anger and may experience distressing nightmares or memories. Bass and Davis (1988) write that abuse survivors learn to cope by not allowing themselves to experience these feelings to their full extent and learn not to trust their feelings. 'In essence, the traumatised person often survives by forfeiting her own voice' (Austin 2002, p.234).

There is an established body of knowledge clearly linking a history of child abuse with higher rates in adult life of depressive symptoms, anxiety symptoms, substance abuse disorders, eating disorders and traumatic stress disorders (Mullen *et al.* 1996). Adult survivors may have difficulties in communicating, as it has not been safe to do so as a child, and their developmental capacity for trust, intimacy, agency and sexuality may be impacted upon. Survivors of childhood sexual abuse may also experience low self-esteem, suicidal ideation and poor body image (Clendenon-Wallen 1991).

Rationale for using songwriting with this population

The group songwriting process described in this chapter developed from collaborative work with a social work colleague. She became aware within her role as family support worker facilitating parenting support programmes that many of the parents with whom she was working had not healed from their traumatic experiences as children. None of the parents involved in the programmes had experienced unconditional love as children. Generational deficits in parenting had been passed on, so that there was often no clear notion of nurturing. For many of these women, there was a hurting child within.

O'Brien (1991) writes of the need to make parenting programmes for vulnerable parents therapeutic as well as educative and discussed several important aspects of working with this client population. First, programmes need to address the lack of trust clients may have of others which can be achieved within a group context by establishing ground rules and clear expectations about attendance etc. Second, clients may have the opportunity to release themselves from their hurtful pasts so that they can move on to incorporating new approaches in parenting their children. O'Brien (1991) describes that enhancing parents' self-esteem and sense of control is vital in allowing them to effectively take charge of their lives. The important aspects of therapeutic and educative programmes, as outlined by O'Brien, are inherent in the songwriting process.

Smyth (2002) discusses creativity as central to the process of healing from trauma as a way of overcoming helplessness. 'Creating something new is an act of defiance in the face of destruction' (Smyth 2002, p.76). Since songwriting is a

What rebonds ⟨

creative act, it can be seen as a way of promoting many of the healing qualities inherent in creative acts (Schmidt 1983). It has also been described as effective in achieving goals such as group cohesiveness, increasing self-expression and self-esteem, improving interpersonal communication, recovering repressed material and enhancing insight into personal issues (Edgerton 1990). It is for these reasons, and with the aim of helping women to find their voices after enduring a lifetime of silence and secrecy, that this method of songwriting was developed.

Many of the women involved in my songwriting programmes have endured abuse throughout their childhoods and into their adult years. Their lives are often chaotic, oppressed by both violence and poverty and in many cases they have been marginalized from mainstream society. Many have had poor educational opportunities and have extremely low self-confidence and an inability to trust both themselves and their significant others. All have experienced at least one form of childhood abuse and many have experienced all forms, such as physical, emotional, psychological, sexual, neglect and exposure to family violence.

Methodological orientation

The songwriting programmes discussed in this chapter employ an eclectic music therapy methodology based on humanistic and feminist theories. They also utilize the 'strengths perspective framework' (Saleebey 2002) and incorporate the concepts of social justice such as access, equity, rights and participation (Jones and May 1997), which promote inclusiveness and respectfulness. A supportive group therapy model was adopted to enhance the intrinsic therapeutic qualities of groups, e.g. normalization and cohesion (Yalom 1995), and enhance the strengths of the group members in coping with their past traumas (Foy, Eriksson and Trice 2001). Foy *et al.* write that supportive group therapy places little attention on the details of the traumatic events, instead preferring to focus on the validation of the impact of the trauma experience on group members' daily lives.

The feminist principles underpinning the work include empowerment, inclusiveness and the breaking down of power dichotomies. Feminist counselling approaches emphasize collaboration which values the competence of both client and worker and respects the client's choices as to what point and in what way she wants to talk about her experiences (Palmer 1991). As Rogers (2003) states, addressing issues of power is highly important when working with survivors of abuse 'as abuse, by its very nature, is about power within relationships in which one (usually larger and stronger, embodied with more authority) uses their power to exploit another (usually smaller, weaker and embodied with less authority)' (Rogers 2003, p.135).

The programmes

In contrast to much music therapy work, where songwriting may be offered to clients as only one technique that forms a part of the music therapy process, the work described here involves songwriting as the major therapeutic technique. Clients self-refer to programmes with the knowledge that they are songwriting programmes aimed at addressing issues relating to childhood abuse experiences. Clients are parents who are aiming to stop the cycle of violence perpetuating to their own children. They are seeking a greater awareness of the impact of their abuse on their parenting and their ability to cope as adults.

Programmes run over a series of 12 weeks culminating in the recording of the clients' song creations upon conclusion. Feedback from focus group research data indicates that this is an adequate amount of time for clients to feel connected to the group, to learn to trust group members and programme facilitators and to feel comfortable expressing feelings, thoughts and beliefs. A group format is utilized as it is thought that clients gain much from the support of other women who have experienced similar childhood circumstances. Workshops are held weekly for two hours and typically include the sharing of morning or afternoon tea. Groups are purposefully small in size, usually between four and eight members. It is explained at the commencement of the workshops that attendance on a weekly basis wherever possible is required to allow for a consistent group membership.

On the first day of the workshop series, clients are introduced to the concept of music therapy and songwriting and the process is explained. I explain that many people find the use of music and songwriting helpful in expressing feelings and memories and discuss a little of what my role is in facilitating the creation of songs. In some instances an example of a previous group song is played to clients so that they may have a clearer idea of what the group might achieve. It is identified at the outset that it is OK if the group does not complete a song over the course of the 12 weeks to minimize the pressure potentially experienced by clients. The emphasis in describing the songwriting process is placed on the sharing of ideas, thoughts and feelings, and working through solutions with other group members.

A warm-up to the discussions is facilitated by encouraging clients to bring in recorded music that has personal significance to them and to share this music with the group. These song choices are generally shared with the group at the commencement and conclusion of workshops and are effective in developing group cohesion. In addition, this task is useful as it allows the music therapist to become familiar with the range of preferred styles of music within the group membership.

As a result of childhood abuse, adult survivors often feel like they are not believed. It is imperative to this work that each group member's opinions, feelings and experiences are validated and listened to. Throughout the songwriting process it is vital to give each participant the chance to be heard and their voice to be represented within the words of the song.

It is important to include two facilitators when working with groups containing individuals who have such complex needs. This allows for one facilitator to continue with the group and its momentum while the other attends to individuals if they become distressed and require individual support. The combination of two facilitators from different disciplines further allows for multiple observations and interpretations of client participation, as well as professional support in attuning to the needs of the group. Having two facilitators also provides opportunities for peer debriefing which is both valuable and necessary.

The method

The steps involved in this particular songwriting method are as follows:

- weeks 1–4: brainstorming on themes including:
  - effect of childhood abuse on the clients and their children
  - self-esteem
  - anger
  - trust
  - domestic violence and its impact on children
  - social isolation
  - rights of children
  - verbal abuse and its impact on children's self-worth
  - communicating positively with children and significant others
  - self-harm, body image and suicide
  - managing stress and relaxation techniques
- weeks 5–7: lyric creation
- weeks 8–10: creating the music
- weeks 10–12: rehearsing and recording.

It is acknowledged that although this is generally the process undertaken by the group, programme facilitators need to be flexible to the needs of group members and these timelines are not always strictly adhered to. A group may also want to create more than one song and as a result may take longer to complete any one of the stages. The following are descriptions of what is typically involved in these four stages of the songwriting process.

Step one: brainstorming on themes

During the initial stages of the programmes, clients are encouraged, through participating in group discussions, to contribute thoughts and feelings around identified issues and themes. They are also invited to suggest issues and themes that they would like to explore further in the group context. These topics are specifically chosen by the facilitators as a starting point in formulating ideas for the song due to their prevalence within the documented experiences of abused women. During this process, participants' responses are recorded on butcher's paper and then typed up at the conclusion of each workshop ready for presentation to the group the following week. This aspect of the method is important because it allows for confirmation that the clients' contributions were recorded accurately, it refreshes clients' memories on recent discussions and provides a starting point for continuing the discussions. Generally, this process takes around the first three to four weeks of the group.

Step two: lyric creation

The next stage of this songwriting process focuses on developing the lyrics for the group's songs. This stage involves the following steps:

1.   identifying the key issues/themes the group feels are most important for inclusion in their songs

2.   further discussion on these themes

3.   identifying a main idea/theme for the chorus

4.   putting together the brainstorming from these issues into a song structure – identifying chorus theme and additional verse lyrics.

A more traditional verse/chorus song outline is most often offered, as it is believed to be the format with which most group members are familiar, according to their musical styles and preferences. As the chorus is often repeated throughout the song it is identified as containing the key issue for the group at that moment. In this way the topic chosen by the group on which to base the chorus may serve as an evaluation tool in establishing into what issues or feelings group members may require further exploration. Much discussion around lyric generation takes place in the group context. It has also been common for group members to write their own verses on the group themes for inclusion in the song.

All group members are given a sketchpad and a notebook at the beginning of each series of workshops and encouraged to write or draw on the days between each workshop if they feel they want to. Group members are encouraged to share their recorded ideas or drawings with each other. Many clients have commented that this assists them to process some of what is discussed within the group context. They have also described this technique as helpful in that many feelings and memories emerge at odd times such as in the middle of the night when there is no possibility of sharing these thoughts and feelings with others. In these situations, they can use the pen and paper to write down these ideas which can then be taken to the group at the next session.

Once the group has decided what they want to include in their songs, the music therapist presents them with several options for lyrical content. Group members then discuss and decide which options best reflect the nature of what they want to say. Careful attention is paid to not changing any of the clients' words, and if words do have to be changed to fit the structure of the song more closely, this is done within the group context and agreed upon by all group members.

Step three: creating the music

During step 3, the songs really start to take a musical form. This process most often involves the following:

- decisions on melodic and accompaniment styles, and tonality as modelled by the music therapist (chord progressions and melodic suggestions are most often created by the music therapist rather than the clients themselves)

- decisions on genre of song – group members may have an artist or style of song already in mind for their words

- decisions on instrumentation – that is, does it need keyboard/guitar accompaniment or inclusion of drum kit/other instruments to reflect the nature of the feeling contained within the song?

- therapist-provided choices to clients incorporating their decisions on song styles

- group decision on which choice best reflects and supports their lyrical content.

As most group members have had no prior musical experience, this can be a very daunting process. My initial thoughts on working with this client group were that they would have a more active role in making music for the songs. These thoughts were quickly turned around, however, when I saw the fear in many of their faces at the suggestion of picking up an instrument or humming a melody. Most of the women involved in these projects have such poor senses of self-esteem that any suggestion of active music-making with the chance of perhaps not succeeding was out of the question. When offered, they were very comfortable with making choices and directing the music creation, but were not at all comfortable with making the music no matter how much reassurance and facilitation I gave as the therapist. Many commented: 'That is what you are here for.' In cases where I have facilitated individuals writing their own songs (outside of the group context), more input on the creation of the music was often possible.

With initial versions of the songs completed, generally around week 9 of the programme, there are opportunities to refine and change aspects of the song with which clients are not satisfied. This is always an exciting part of the process as the clients begin to take more ownership of their songs. Clients will often tell me if they find something too boring, too high to sing, too fast etc. and many have had lengthy discussions around changing as little as one word. It is believed important for the therapist to let the group work through these decisions, however frustrating this might be at the time. I recall one conversation lasting 45 minutes about whether the word 'that' was needed at the beginning of a line in the song. This particular part of the process is often very empowering and important for clients as they search to find the exact words to describe their experiences. Minor adjustments to the music are also called for; however, generally by week 10 of the programme, songs will be completed.

Step four: rehearsing and recording

Group members are involved in rehearsing and recording their creations during the final weeks of the programme. By this stage, even those group members who stated at the commencement of the programme that they would definitely not sing are generally starting to sing their words. Decisions are made on who is going to sing and whether or not the group requires assistance from the therapist or whether they feel confident enough to sing on their own. For those who are still finding it difficult to find their voices, the music therapist will often suggest that a spoken part be included in the song so that they would still have involvement. This technique is effective in allowing all group members to be involved at their own level. At times, whole songs may involve spoken verses and sung choruses, at the request of group members.

Although the programme does not emphasize the importance of rehearsing, as the essence of the programme is not to achieve a 'perfect' product, what is important is that group members feel comfortable and familiar with their involvement prior to the recording session. It is also at this time that the group cohesion is strong as the clients become aware that they have achieved something together. There are often tears and much laughter during this rehearsing time as all the emotion that has been put into creating the songs comes to the fore.

On the recording day, the therapist should record musical tracks and a vocal guide if required for clients to sing along to prior to the arrival of the group. Enlisting the help of colleagues (at the permission of group members) to provide additional musical support when the song calls for it is often valuable. This is all completed before the women arrive so that all our attention can be focused on them. The recording session is considered to be an extremely important part of this songwriting process as clients 'beam' with pride when they hear their songs recorded.

In follow-up research interviews, many clients have commented that this recording process was a highlight for them. Words of one participant seem to sum up the general feelings of clients:

> Standing behind that microphone, singing those words, it was great, honestly felt I didn't want to walk out of there, I wanted to stay there…standing there like you are a music star…it was great mate…we'd actually done it mate…you know…us bunch of girls had the feelings about ourselves that we couldn't really see anything through and we'd actually done it…and we'd done a bloody good job of it too…we were pretty impressed…pretty proud of ourselves!

Although the songs often contain extremely emotive and painful material, clients cope well with this on the recording day. They have indicated that through the songwriting process itself, from beginning to discuss their feelings to working through changing words and rehearsing their songs, their painful stories are externalized and feelings relating to their childhood experiences become more neutral. The excitement and strong sense of doing something important for themselves and others may also contribute to overcoming the emotional content of their songs.

Clients have commented that it was extremely important to have their songs recorded as it provided a tangible outcome from the workshops – 'the closing of a book', in one participant's words. It is for this reason that the recording stage is included as a step in the songwriting process. Creating songs and recording them on CD has been described as a way of making something positive out of all their negative experiences.

Group members have gone on to share their songs with loved ones, friends and their children and have been invited to present their songs at numerous functions including violence prevention conferences and forums. They share them with people to create a greater understanding of where it is that their difficulties may stem from. Clients have felt that it is important to present their songs, however emotional it may be for them, as a way of raising awareness in the community of the impact of childhood abuse. In this way the process has taken on a social action role, something that I would like to explore further as an aspect to this work.

Case example: 'Living a lie'

To illustrate the songwriting method I employ with women who have experienced abuse, I have selected one song written by a group of four women and describe its creation and recording process, step by step. Of these four women, two had experienced childhood sexual assault, and the other two had experienced physical and psychological violence as children. The average age of the clients was 32. One of the group members had not previously spoken about her abuse with others for fear of being judged. In writing their song, they communicated a clear message to society and particularly to health professionals. Their song was entitled 'Living a lie' and speaks of the feelings the women have of keeping up appearances and wearing a mask in society due to their fear of being judged.

Step 1: brainstorming on themes

The themes brainstormed in writing the song during the early part of the programme are listed in Table 4.1.

Step 2: lyric creation

From the initial thoughts and feelings of the group combined with some individual phrases/verses written by group members on the themes, I offered the lyrics below as one suggestion for the group to consider.

LYRICS PRESENTED TO GROUP MEMBERS
I always felt like a little adult as a child
Home is your refuge, your safe haven so we're told
I need to make it safe and tell the world the truth
That I wasn't even safe under my own roof

The things that happen you don't see
Are hidden by our/my masks
Some people look at me and judge for what they see
They need to look behind the mask and see the real me

Table 4.1 Ideas brainstormed for the song 'Living a lie'

Theme	Responses from participants around the themes
Play acting	Not having the skills to live life Never being sure you are playing the right role Keeping up appearances/wearing a mask Keeping your face up to the outside world Not very good to spend a lifetime not expressing your emotions Home is your cubby hole, your safe haven
Society	Not feeling a part of mainstream society People think they have the right to judge Money plays a part in outcomes People not listening – don't want to know Health professionals don't listen either – they want to give you medication Only now feeling like an adult
Self-esteem	Always felt like a 'little adult' as a child Always struggling to improve Never feeling like you've got it together Caught in a frustrating cycle Spent a lifetime abusing myself, so I don't have to deal with it Never had the opportunities to express myself
Family	Learning inappropriate things from your family about sex and relationships Loss of family/family unit now so small Whole family picture was a lie
Child protection	Protecting kids Watching and wondering if you're doing the same things to your kids as was done to you – have to change that Want children to be educated
Impact of abuse	Lifetime of sadness Taught not to listen to your instincts When you live with abuse it teaches you to accept the unacceptable Nowhere was safe Scared of going outside Memories – like ghosts haunting As a child you don't have a choice Bashing your head against a brick wall Anger, despair – no-one to talk to Everything comes at a cost
Additional themes	No avenue for help, no-one to walk hand-in-hand with you Other forms of therapy – 'time's up' – takes too long to get to what you want to talk about

Society only wants to see the functioning side of me
You're not interested in the/my pain and trauma
That lives inside of me

You prefer me to play a role
Take 3 pills and call me/go away
You don't really hear anything I say
Just conform and get on with it/deal with it
'There there, it will all go away'
It doesn't go, it's always there
To haunt us once again
It's a part of your life that you won't forget/can't go away
Reminders of those times will always filter through
No matter where you go, no matter what you do

You're told you don't know what you're feeling
And learn not to trust your own instincts
You don't listen to yourself, everyone else 'knows better'
Keeps you in the cycle of abuse

From this point, group members discussed what the most important theme was for a chorus. They decided that they wanted their song to rhyme and that the main thing they wanted to say to society was that people needed to listen more. They chose a verse–chorus–verse–chorus structure and set about choosing which lines they wanted to keep and those which they wanted to reword or rephrase. At this stage the musical elements of the song were introduced so that the fine-tuning of the lyrics could be made according to the rhythm of the melody.

Step 3: creating the music

I offered group members choices of various melodic and accompaniment styles. Clients chose the key of E minor for their song as they felt it reflected the feeling within the song and suited their vocal ranges. They wanted a strong rhythmical guitar accompaniment rather than a picking accompaniment and decided on the tempo of the song. Changes were made to the lyrics to fit with the melody they chose and group members started to sing along with their song.

The first verse and chorus in the final version of the song can be seen in Figure 4.1 and the lyrics in full are detailed below.

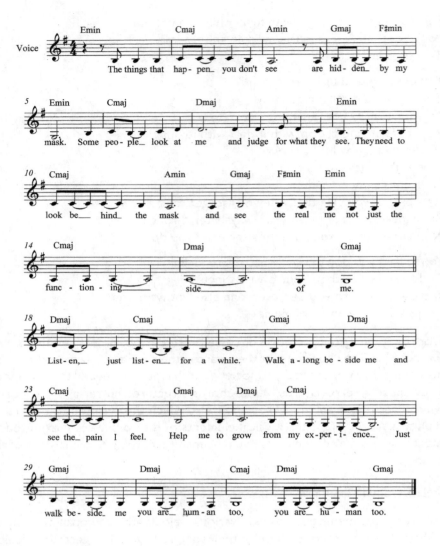

Figure 4.1 'Living a lie'

FINAL VERSION OF THE LYRICS TO 'LIVING A LIE'

The things that happen you don't see
Are hidden by my mask
Some people look at me and
Judge for what they see
They need to look behind the mask
And see the real me
Not just the functioning
Side of me

Listen, just listen for a while
Walk along beside me and see the pain I feel
Help me to grow from my experience
Just walk beside me, you are human too.

You're not interested in the pain
That lives inside my veins
You prefer me to play a role
Being happy, being whole
You think you can label me, but hear
Nothing that I say
Take these pills and call me
Just conform or go away

I always felt like a little adult as a child
Home should be your refuge, your safe haven so we're told
I need to make it safe and tell the world the truth
That I wasn't even safe under my own roof.

This ghost in my life
I can't escape
Will haunt me once again
Part of my life I can't forget
Reminders of those times
Will always filter through
No matter where I go
No matter what I do

I just need you to listen, just listen for a while
Walk along beside me and see the pain I feel
Help me to grow from my experience
Just walk beside me you are human too, you are human too.

Concluding remarks

It is suggested, then, that this method of therapeutic songwriting can assist in meeting the needs of adults who have experienced childhood trauma by achieving the following goals:

- developing or enhancing clients' sense of self-esteem and sense of identity

- facilitating the expression of feelings around painful childhood experiences within a group context

- gaining validation for feelings and experiences from facilitators and peer group
- identifying the impact of abuse on themselves and their children
- providing opportunities for empowerment through choice
- development of the ability to trust both themselves and significant others.

I have discussed important considerations for music therapy clinicians throughout this chapter. I reiterate that it is important to work within a multi-disciplinary team and have agencies to refer to at the completion of such a programme if follow-up support is required. It is vital for the group to have as much choice in the creation of their songs as possible and that all feelings and thoughts are represented and acknowledged within the songwriting process. It is also useful to explain to group members at the outset (especially when there are children residing with clients) the mandates and processes we have as health practitioners in reporting child abuse in the event of disclosures within the group.

Remaining open and empathic to the stories of women, believing those stories and facilitating the finding of clients' voices through therapeutic songwriting appears to assist survivors of childhood abuse in providing closure, beginning healing and providing hope for the future for themselves and their families.

Note

Acknowledgements go to the many women who have shared their stories and allowed me to share in their personal journeys through songwriting processes and to my inspirational colleague Helen Bruderer who has contributed significantly to the development of this songwriting method.

5

Collaborations on Songwriting with Clients with Mental Health Problems

Randi Rolvsjord

This chapter will focus on songwriting in individual music therapy with adult clients with mental health problems. With my own clinical practice as a starting point, I will describe the role of songwriting as one possible and useful musical interaction with clients. I will present a set of techniques for collaborating with clients when creating both song lyrics and melodies. These techniques will be exemplified through a case presentation, which will also illustrate the therapeutic function of songwriting.

In my work in a psychiatric hospital, songwriting has emerged as a form of musical interaction that I frequently employ with my clients in individual sessions of music therapy. I believe there are at least three reasons for this. The first reason is that song is a very familiar and a commonly used musical form in the Norwegian culture, as it is in many other cultures. Thus, most people I meet in my practice already have a degree of competence related to songs. They have a large repertoire of popular songs and folk songs which they know well, and they are familiar with the most typical verse–refrain structures. They have prior experience that songs can be used in different ways and for different reasons and that some songs are particularly meaningful to them. It seems that for many of the patients I meet, singing and playing songs is a type of musical interaction in which they easily and naturally let themselves become engaged. When songs are the starting point for musical interaction in music therapy, writing songs is just a small step away.

Writing songs is also a musical activity and interaction which I really enjoy and find very useful in therapy. Because of this I will often suggest writing songs as a way of working, and I will go into such activity with a lot of involvement which motivates the client to continue. I think my own pleasure and interest in writing

...important, but, in addition, I think that the songwriting activity has specific ...entials for providing important emotional relational experiences. Emotional involvement is inevitably part of any musical interaction, but in the process of songwriting this is explicated within the song product. In songwriting, the participants will make use of their musical and poetic skills, will use their musical identity and knowledge of different musical genres, and express their emotions related to the theme of the song. The role and function of songwriting will vary according to the music therapeutic process as a whole. There are, however, some general aspects of songs that might provide some understanding of why songwriting seems to be meaningful in therapy:

- Songs are a common form of expression.
- Songs can be performed over and over again.
- Songs can be shared.
- Songs can be kept and stored away.

Songwriting in therapy consists of a process of creating the song and all the musical, verbal and bodily communication involved in that process. As Trygve Aasgaard has pointed to in his doctoral dissertation (Aasgaard 2002), the therapeutic process concerned with songwriting does not end when the song is finished. The process evolves further once the product is achieved. The therapeutic process, with the product, continues as the song is rehearsed with different instruments (Rolvsjord 2001), as the song is sung repeatedly in therapy, as the song is performed for other therapists, family or friends, or sometimes even performed in concert (Aasgaard 2002; Aigen 2004). The meaning of a song, and the therapeutic potentials of songwriting in music therapy then, is not only connected to the song as a certain expression, but to the relational experiences of the songwriting process and to the use of the song inside and outside the music therapy room.

Songwriting with clients with mental health problems

Adult clients with mental health problems are a very heterogeneous group of clients both related to their problems and illnesses, to their resources, and musical competence and skills. Their musical and verbal competence, capacity and skills connected to songwriting vary in approximately the same way as for the rest of the adult population. Mental illness is explained according to various biological, sociological or psychological models. In most cases, however, the causes of the condition are disputed or unknown (Mechanic 1999). Consequently the different models have resulted in the development of different types of treatment, medical as well as psychotherapeutic, but in most cases the most effective treatment is uncertain (Lambert and Ogles 2004; Mechanic 1999; Wampold 2001). Further, to work in mental health is to work with a population with very different needs, different problems and different levels of functioning. Thus clients seem to make use of different types of therapeutic interventions, not only in relation to the diagnostic variations, but also according to their resources, such as interests, personal coping skills, social network and culture, etc. (Duncan and Miller 2000; Tallman and Bohart 1999).

I take a resource-oriented approach in my clinical work with clients with mental health problems (Rolvsjord 2003). A resource-oriented approach is strongly connected to empowerment philosophy (Rolvsjord 2004) and involves some central aims and philosophies:

- to amplify strengths rather than to mend weaknesses of the clients
- to recognize competencies related to their therapeutic process of change
- to nurture and develop the resources of clients through musical interactions and collaborations in the therapeutic process
- to focus on musical resources and music as resource.

In general, clients are referred to music therapy for two reasons. First, clients are referred because they have an interest in music or they might be interested in music. Second, clients are referred because they are not motivated or assessed as not suitable for verbal psychotherapy. According to the principles of the resource-oriented approach, I recognize clients' knowledge about their needs and about how music can be useful for them inside and outside therapy. Consequently, songwriting is preferred when clients regard this as a useful way of working. Usually songwriting is used with clients who are observed to express themselves through songs, and/or with clients that have musical or poetic skills that they want to develop.

The usefulness of songwriting in a therapeutic process might first of all be connected to the songs as a narrative, to the expression and communication of feelings and experiences (Ficken 1976; Nolan 1998; Rolvsjord 2001; Smith 1991), as well as to the expression and communication of cultural identity through the choices of musical genres and styles (McFerran in press). Second, songwriting in therapy might provide experiences of mastery related to the skills demonstrated in songwriting. The development of such musical skills can be considered part of cultural capital important for the client's sense of self-esteem and self-efficacy, but also related to his/her participation in communities.

Method and techniques of songwriting

As described above, the resource-oriented approach implies that client and therapist are collaborating in the therapeutic process and that the client's competence is recognized in the way he or she uses music. Therefore, when I meet a new client, I might suggest different ways of working, including writing songs as a possibility for our musical interaction, and start with songwriting if the client is interested.

There are probably as many ways of writing songs as there are songwriters. I think of a song as having lyrics, a melody and most often a harmonic progression and a quite simple form. One example is the verse–refrain form. The process of writing a song could start with either of these parts, but will in most cases involve a dynamic and flexible play with melody, lyrics and harmony. Most typically, the lyrics, or at least some verbal givens, are the starting point for the song creations, but other times the songs may develop from an improvisation with or without words. I do not have a rigid procedure in my method of songwriting, but adjust the method to the client's skills and resources. If the client is already writing poems, these are a natural starting point. Other times the client has come up with a musical theme, a melody or a composition that looks like a song, or an improvisation we made has some themes that could be developed into a song. When we have a starting point or an idea for the song, the rest is a process of adapting melody to lyrics, lyrics to melody, elaborating on the different harmonies to create an atmosphere that fits the melody and lyrics, and creating the musical form that is a song.

The most common form of songs is probably the verse–refrain structure, or the even more simple structure of verse following a similar verse. However, at times, it may be difficult to adapt the verbal and musical material into such a strict structure and including a bridge within the song, or a tag at the end is useful to adapt the musical form to the lyrics (O'Brien 2004). In Norwegian vocal folk music tradition, it is common to repeat the fourth, or the second and the fourth phrase of a verse in all other verses within the song. In my clinical work with songwriting, this traditional form is sometimes adapted and used in a more popular-music style.

The process of songwriting may take between one and three sessions, which includes some homework for the therapist, the client or both. I always transcribe the song onto manuscript paper, and make a recording of the song that the client can take away with them. The musical notation (melody, chords and lyrics) is sometimes important in assisting the client in learning to play the song and also makes it possible for other people to play the song. In addition it creates a concrete musical product which can be stored and retrieved at a later date. I give the client the copyright of the song and ask for permission to use the songs outside music therapy. The client is free to use the songs in any way they choose.

Co-creations of lyrics

Through my work with this population, I have developed a number of strategies that are useful in aiding the creation of lyrics.

Technique 1: selecting words from a list of words

Sometimes clients find it hard to express themselves using verbal language. One strategy which I have used to address this is to create a list of words from which the clients can select specific words that they think should be included in a song. I create this list of words and symbols from stories the clients have shared and from songs we have sung or listened to within the therapy sessions (Rolvsjord 2001).

Technique 2: client self-generates words

When I suggest to clients that we could create a song together, I often suggest that they could write down a few words on a piece of paper that they might want to include in the song. When I go on and make a song based upon such a list of words, or some sentences, I will try to make the lyrics as open and poetic as possible in order to make sure that several interpretations of the song are possible so that the client can fill the song with his or her own meaning (Rolvsjord 2001).

Technique 3: client writes a poem

Sometimes clients contribute their material in the form of a poem. In these situations, the exact wording in the poem is not always identical with the lyrics in the final product of the song. Sometimes some words are deleted or added in order to adapt to the song melody. Other times one part of the poem is repeated (for example as a refrain) to conform to a particular musical form.

Co-creations of songs from clients' poems

When clients bring poems into music therapy with the purpose of transforming them into songs, I usually ask the client about the poem: their themes, emotions, situations and the experiences that they express. Then I try to find out from the client if he or she has any thoughts about how the music should sound – focusing on parameters such as genre, tonality, tempo, etc. From here, the song is created through the use of three different basic techniques, or a combination of these:

- therapist creates melody between therapy sessions
- therapist creates melody within the therapy session
- therapist and client improvise melodies together.

Technique 1: therapist creates melody between sessions

The therapist might create a song out of the poem between the sessions and present it to the client at the following session. Any suggestion from the client according to genre, chords or form needs to be taken into consideration. When I have created a melody between the sessions it is usually just because the poem is 'crying' for a melody and then suddenly I have an idea which is put down on a sheet of paper. Sometimes it seems too difficult for the client to go into the theme of the song. To help the client not to be overwhelmed by the emotions expressed in the song, or even re-traumatized by the exposure, I find that creating the melody between the sessions can be a way of regulating the focus upon such very difficult emotions and traumatic experiences.

When I bring the song with me at the next session, I always present it as a sug-gestion or an idea that could be further developed or rejected and often present alter-natives to the client. Obviously this is not always an appropriate technique to use as this could be understood by some clients as an implicit devaluation of their skills, or even a theft of their poem. Pointing to the poetic skills of the client can be a way of reducing the risk of clients experiencing this feeling. At other times this can be a very appropriate approach, and be a confirmation of the collaboration and the thera-pist's commitment in the therapeutic process. When the therapist creates the song out of the poem, she also shares some of her responses (interpretations, associations and emotions), as expressed in the music with the client. Such an emotional rela-tional experience might be very useful for the client in order to achieve contact and insight into his/her emotions, as you will see exemplified through the case example later in the chapter.

Technique 2: therapist creates melody within the therapy session

It is often in the therapeutic interests of the clients to be actively engaged in creating the music. To facilitate this, I may start to improvise and come up with some ideas for melody and harmonic progressions. The client is encouraged to come forward with her own ideas, or to accept or reject my suggestions. To achieve this, I may offer alternative melodies, ask the clients for advice, and ask for feedback regarding the different harmonic or rhythmic patterns I may try out.

Technique 3: therapist and client improvise melodies together

This third technique is inspired by Diana Austin's vocal holding techniques (Austin 1999, 2002). We start by finding a simple harmonic pattern that creates an atmosphere appropriate to the theme communicated within the lyrics. Usually I suggest a two-chord pattern, but sometimes a four-chord pattern, depending upon the character of the lyrics and the musical and improvisational competencies of the client. We begin with a little warm-up exercise to become familiar with the harmonic scheme. Then we start improvising, and take turns in singing every second phrase. We continue with this until some part of the song takes shape. At this point, I musically notate the phrases to avoid forgetting them. Sometimes we find that the song would benefit from some harmonic variations to avoid monotony and this can be achieved by adding a different harmonic pattern within the song, for example during the refrain.

Case example: Emma's songs

To illustrate and exemplify these songwriting techniques and the role of songwriting in the process of music therapy, I will introduce you to the story about a young woman, whom I will call Emma, and our work in music therapy. The story and the songs are presented with kind permission from the client.

Emma is a young woman in her early twenties. She is a survivor of severe childhood abuse. Growing up in a home with a mentally ill mother and a violent father, she has experienced a trauma which lasted for about 20 years of her life, and she is suffering from post-traumatic stress disorder due to these experiences. In spite of her hard life she has managed to finish secondary school and had started tertiary education at the time I first met her. She was actively involved in organizations and had good contact with friends. She was admitted to the psychiatric hospital in order to work with her trauma within the safe frames of a hospitalization. She started in music therapy because she was interested in music and her first goal in music therapy was to start singing again. She told me that singing had been a very important part of her life, but that singing had more and more become related to performance anxiety, and that she had gradually stopped singing and now was afraid that her voice was ugly.

In the beginning sessions we mainly sang together, and after a short while she was able to sing out loud again. After a few sessions I suggested to her that we also could write our own songs, and that a beginning for this could be for her to write down a few words and sentences to bring to her next session. From then on she started to bring poems that she had written about her feelings and experiences to music therapy sessions, and we started to create songs together. After 16 months within the hospital, Emma was discharged but music therapy outpatient sessions continued. After two-and-a-half years of working together, we had created more than 30 songs, based upon her poems. In parallel with the songwriting, we continued to sing pre-composed songs together and to talk about the songs and the feelings and meanings they represented for her. Some of the song lyrics explicitly tell stories about her traumas. Other songs communicate feelings of loneliness, despair and anxiety, but some also express wishes and hopes.

The songs I present in the following sections illustrate different ways of creating songs, which have served different functions within Emma's therapeutic process. The fourth song created within Emma's music therapy programme was entitled 'Father's crime'.

Father's crime
little and scared
always filled with fear
because of a father's hand
whose touching so often it can

struggling and fighting
against the world of pain whose biting
father's lips touch
and the pain is just too much

living and dying
what to choose, or maybe crying
father's hand stole your soul
and made the world around you so cold

Emma brought this poem into music therapy in her ninth session and we used the following three sessions to complete the song. The lyrics were originally written in English and were not changed during the process of creating the song, except for the repetition of the last strophe/sentence in the last verse. Although she brought the poem to session 9, we did not start to work on the song's melodic line until the following session (session 10). In the days following session 10, I created a song out of the poem, and presented this for her in the following session. During session 11, the song was finally finished and Emma gave the song the title 'Father's crime'. The final version of the song is illustrated in Figure 5.1.

Constructing a melody for a song inevitably implies that you involve yourself emotionally, and the melody will express some of your own feelings connected to the lyrics. It so happened in this song that there was a discrepancy between the musical expression of the song which I had created and Emma's emotions and anticipations of the musical effect. I had created her song within a rock 'n' roll genre and when she listened to the song for the first time she was surprised

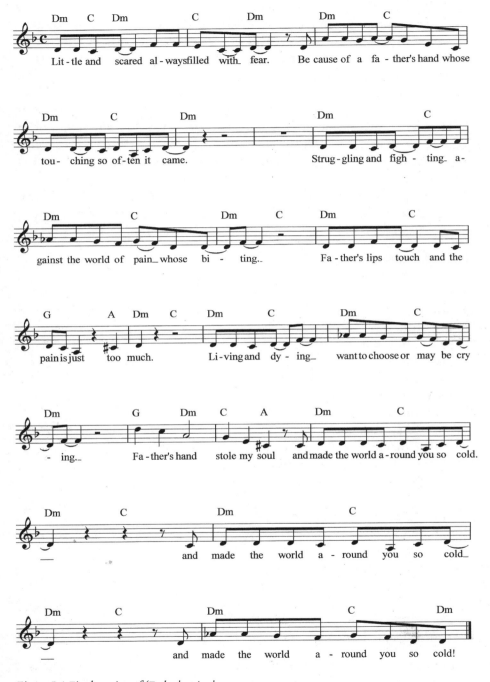

Figure 5.1 Final version of 'Father's crime'

that I had created such an angry song out of her sad lyrics. I told her that I was really feeling very angry about men doing such things to their children, but that we could change the song, if she wanted it to be more a sad song. She then replied, 'Can you make it angrier?' This was achieved not by making any changes to the melody or chords, but through aspects of the performance, such as singing 'on top' of the pulse, accentuating the words 'biting' and 'fighting' and emphasizing the 'blue' notes.

What we can learn here is that the discrepancy between my song creation and her emotions connected to the poem provided for her a new emotional experience. This song, my musical expression of her poem, made it possible for her to get in contact with her anger, and to give her anger an allowable expression through music.

After a difficult period and some hard work with a song exploring Emma's thoughts of suicide, she presented two poems which expressed more positive thoughts and feelings – one of which was 'Cry out and shout'.

Cry out and shout

Cry out and shout
let your voice be heard!
A little girl in a big world
whispering about life that's so heavy
Cry out and shout
let your voice be heard!
A little girl walking down the streets
stumbles, but rising again – quiet
Cry out and shout
let your voice be heard!
Stumbling through life, not complaining
whispering about sorrow and scars in
her mind
Cry out and shout
let your voice be heard!
But no one will listen
no one had time
If you're silent you can hear the little
girl whispering when she stumbles through
her hard life:
Cry out and shout
let your voice be heard!

In the next session, I presented her with an idea for the song's refrain based upon the phrase 'Cry out and shout, let your voice be heard!', which was repeated several times in the poem. We decided to repeat the phrase to let it fit into the form of a refrain, and tried out different alternatives of the second phrase (Figure 5.2).

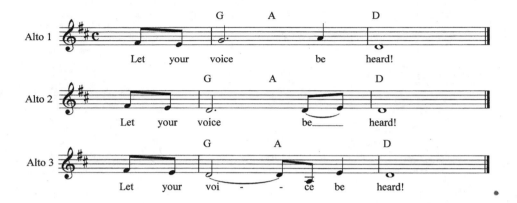

Figure 5.2 Alternatives for the end of the refrain

The alternatives given were quite similar to my original suggestion and had minor importance for the overall structure of the song. The importance of these alternatives is connected to relational aspects of the therapeutic process. These alternatives were presented to Emma because I was uncertain about which ending to choose, and because she was capable of discussing these options with me. Thus it is an example of collaboration and sharing that constitutes and maintains an equal relationship.

Both of us contributed ideas for the melody of the first verse. Later, we went on to work with the rhythms of the second verse which differed from the first in the number of syllables within its phrases but tried to keep a similar melodic shape. Most of the lyrics were adapted to this verse–refrain structure, with only small differences in melody and rhythm occurring between the different verses. These melodic adaptations are illustrated in the final version of the song (Figure 5.3) when bars 8 and 9 are compared with bars 17 and 18, and again with bars 30 and 31.

The sentence 'But no one will listen, no one had time' did not fit into the verse–refrain structure, so we created a bridge leading on to the last verse of the song so that these important words could remain within the song.

In the research interviews it became clear that her experience with this song is very complex. This is her only poem in which she is not taking the voice of the first person. She seems to be looking at herself from a distance. This distance seemed to be strengthened by the music, in particular the gospel-like style of the refrain, which seems to be a bit more jolly and powerful than her

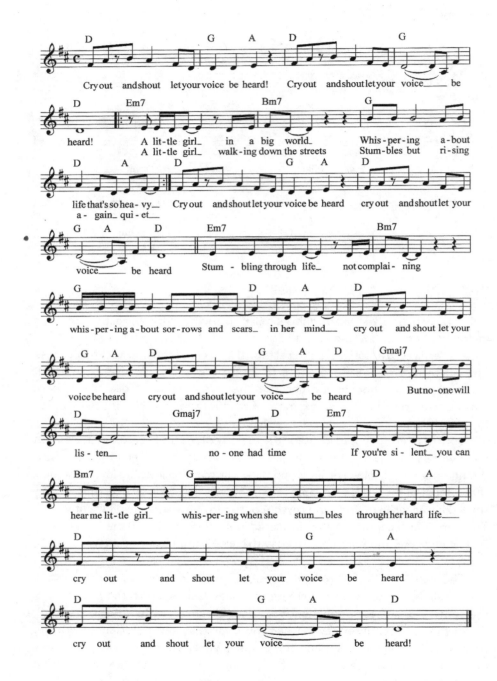

Figure 5.3 Final version of 'Cry out and shout'

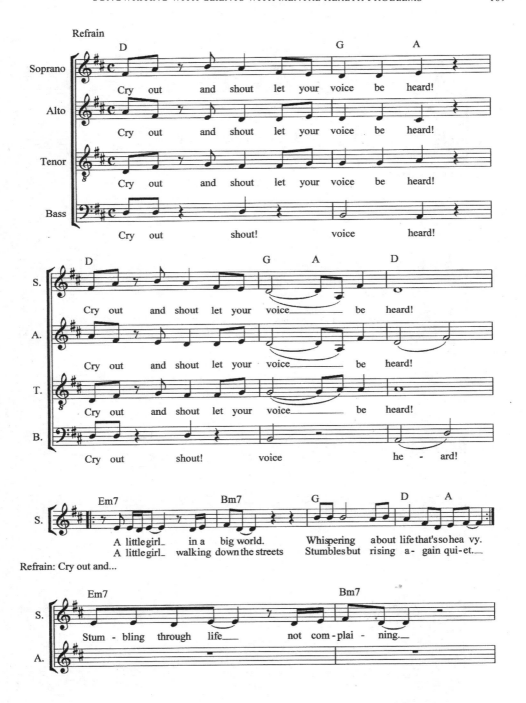

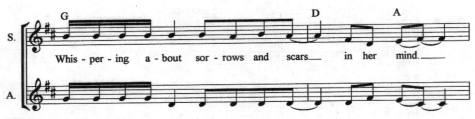

Whis - per - ing a - bout sor - rows and scars___ in her mind.___

Refrain: Cry out and...

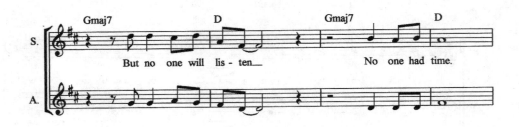

But no one will lis - ten___　　No one had time.

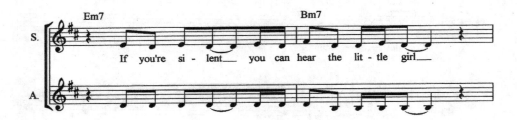

If you're si - lent___ you can hear the lit - tle girl___

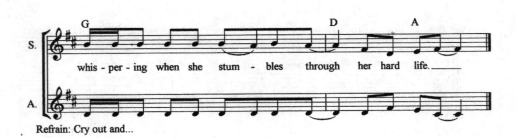

whis - per - ing when she stum - bles through her hard life.___

Refrain: Cry out and...

Figure 5.4 (cont.) 'Cry out and shout' arranged for SATB choir

voice in the poem. But in spite of this distance it seems that this song provides an emotional expression that makes her able to cry out a little bit, at least as long as the song takes to sing.

She has also described this song as the most 'neutral' of the 30 songs which we have created, primarily because of the experienced distance to her own feelings and her identity. This is the only song that she has arranged for a choir and performed in a larger group outside music therapy (Figure 5.4). She explained that the aspect of emotional neutrality and distance in this song made possible for her to experience mastery of musical skills, and through this mastery she regained back a bit of her musical life outside music therapy.

Another poem that Emma wrote was titled 'Be with me now'.

Be with me now

All alone in a world cold as stone
trying to carry it all alone
My life is nothing else than pain,
wish it could be washed away with the rain
But I know it's here to stay,
and I fall on my knees and pray:

Be with me now!
Please, show me when I don't know how
I'm all tired and scared
and my body is filled with fear
Please, don't let me go
be with me now!

I'm trying to survive every day
but it's hard to find the right way
The edge is very near me now
I want to fall down but I don't know how
If I fall there's no more pain,
but I'm too scared to let it rain

As for the technique used for creating a song out of this poem, we used a combination of all the techniques described above. We selected a simple chord progression C–Am–F–G, and started to improvise on every other phrase of the lyrics. After a while some of the phrases began to take form and I wrote down these for us to remember. Then we continued to improvise the sections with which we were not yet happy. This improvisational work resulted in the first part of the verse and an idea for the refrain. In Figure 5.5, I present an example of the improvisation for the first verse. I was improvising the first phrase with the chords C–Am and she would continue with the second phrase with the chords F–G.

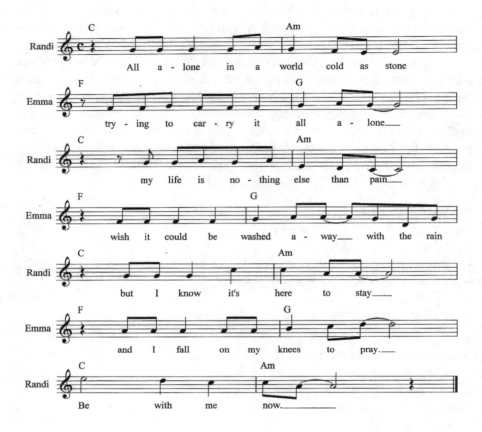

Figure 5.5 Constructed example of the improvisation for the first verse of 'Be with me now'

With this poem, neither of us had a clear idea of a melody. In the turn-taking of the improvisation, an idea evolved as we listened to each other and let ourselves become inspired by each other's expressions. The song developed in a dynamic and mutual interaction of matching and mismatching (Figure 5.6). In the first five phrases there was a lot of matching and a similar contour of the melody was kept. But then in phrase six Emma changed the contour, making a continued upward movement that stimulated me to come up with the distinct motif of the refrain.

After we had decided to use a verse–refrain structure for the song, we worked on the rhythms in the second verse, which were different from those in the first verse. During the third session of working with this song, we created an arrangement with flute.

This song was brought in about two years after her music therapy started. During this period Emma was preparing for her final exams at university. At this

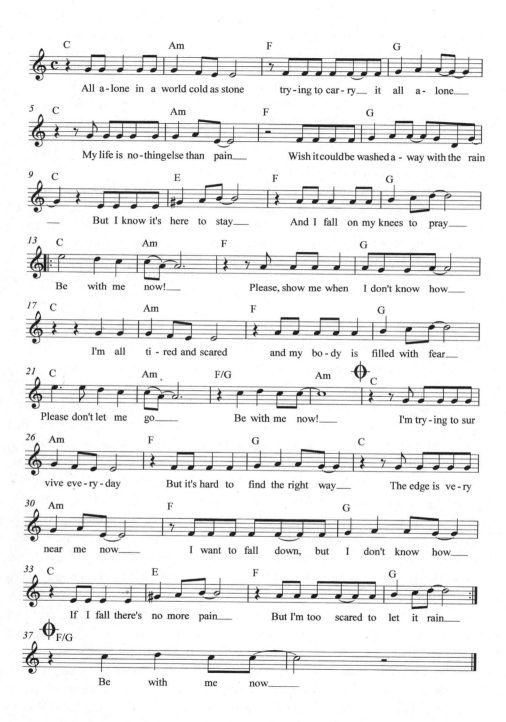

Figure 5.6 The song 'Be with me now'

point there was a lot of uncertainty connected to her future because ending her studies meant that she had to find a job and perhaps a new place to live, and she did not know if it would be possible to continue therapy. In this poem she expresses her loneliness, her need for support, and her anxiety connected to the future and an eventual closure, as well as acknowledging the support she has had from the hospital and the therapists (including me). In the sessions before she brought this poem we talked about the anxiety she felt when people in the hospital commented upon her progress. It seemed like she was very afraid to get well or to manage because she thought that would imply that she would lose all the help and be left alone again.

Two sessions later she invited the psychiatrist to listen to her song, and after that she invited contact from the hospital ward where she stayed on the one day a week she came in for therapy. In an interview she explained that it felt safer to write a song about this theme than to talk about it. But also that after she had sung this song for the psychiatrist and her hospital contact person, she was able to talk with them about her feelings and needs, which resulted in a more clear agreement and announcement of future support from the hospital.

The therapeutic functions of clinical songwriting

As we can see from the three examples from music therapy with Emma, songwriting in music therapy can have very different functions in a therapeutic process. The music sociologist Tia DeNora (2000, 2003) describes musical affordances as a twofold process in which a song or a piece of music has properties or potentials that might become meaningful and useful for people who utilize it. What music affords is dependent upon how it is used. Musical meaning is a product of 'human–music interaction' (DeNora 2003). In this chapter I focused on the therapeutic functions of clinical songwriting based upon the study of this particular case. To understand in what ways songwriting is meaningful in Emma's music therapy, we might look at the songs and the musical expressions of her poems. However, more interesting according to DeNora's theory is how Emma and I interact with the music as we create the songs and how she later uses the songs to work with her feelings and to cope with her life.

Creation of songs is a way of expressing and communicating feelings. Most of Emma's songs are expressions of her emotions connected to different situations and experiences in her life. Sometimes she found that the music had evolved in a different way to that which she had expected. In some cases, as with 'Father's crime', this regulated her emotions and also provided new insight into her own feelings and thoughts. Further, it is important that as expressed in a song, it was possible for her to tolerate the emotions. At other times she experienced that the music confirmed her feelings, and she felt recognized and understood by me. It is also important to note that she found it easier to communicate through the songs than through the verbal language. The songs provided a potential for communication of feelings and thoughts which are too difficult for her to talk about, as with the song 'Be with me now'.

For Emma, her songs were also strongly connected to her identity. Through her songs, she has told the story about her life, her experienced trauma, her feelings, her hopes and wishes. She described the songs as pieces of her, and they all have to be there. In difficult situations she felt that the songs provided something to hold on to, because the songs told her that she had felt a certain way or been in a particular situation before, and that it would not be forever.

Finally writing the songs, as well as playing and singing the songs, is connected to feelings of mastery and joy. She found that her poems, describing horrible experiences and emotions that she did not want to have, could become something beautiful. To experience such positive emotions in musical interaction within music therapy has been important for Emma. Through singing and writing songs, she has regained her rights to music. Songwriting has been an opportunity to show and to further develop some of her musical strengths and resources. She has experienced that she can enjoy music-making again, and she can participate in music-making outside music therapy. Equally important is that the pleasure and joy in music-making has provided a regulation of the intensity of emotions when working with trauma.

6

Songwriting to Explore Identity Change and Sense of Self-concept Following Traumatic Brain Injury

Felicity Baker, Jeanette Kennelly and Jeanette Tamplin

Rehabilitating physical, cognitive and communication functioning following Traumatic Brain Injury (TBI) is an intensive, exhausting and highly emotional task for children, adolescents and adults. Successful rehabilitation relies on clients maintaining high levels of motivation. This is often difficult to achieve, however, when emotional responses to the trauma have an adverse impact on the client's levels of motivation. Over the past 12 years, the authors have successfully employed songwriting interventions with children, adolescents and adult TBI clients to facilitate the adjustment process and to help maintain their motivation for therapy. This chapter will outline the approaches we used in conducting therapeutic songwriting with TBI clients. We first highlight the specific adjustment issues faced by TBI clients to provide a sense of the complexity of dealing with these clients' adjustment processes. Included in this chapter is an explanation of some of the cognitive impairments typically acquired by TBI clients and, more importantly, their impact on the adjustment and songwriting process. Following this, our protocol for writing songs with clients is outlined and this is illustrated through two case examples – one with a late adolescent client and the other with a paediatric client.

Confronting and adjusting to change

Traumatic brain injury is often the outcome of a sudden and unexpected event which results in damage to the brain. Given the unexpected hospitalization and threats to independence, it is not surprising that clients experience emotional crises and often undergo a lengthy adjustment phase. Clients have to adjust and cope with significant life changes that involve accepting many losses: loss of independence and functioning, loss of control, loss of former body, loss of financial status, loss of many roles, loss of future hopes and dreams, and loss of ability to participate in preferred leisure activities.

Several theories have emerged about how and when adjustment occurs and what variables influence the process. Wright (1960) viewed adjustment to disability in terms of it reflecting the interaction between a person's value system, level of emotional maturity and acceptance of self, and mental health status.

Olney and Kim (2001) suggest adjustment is a staged process which includes:

- the response to the initial impact
- defence mobilization
- the initial realization
- a period of retaliation
- reintegration and adjustment which is characterized by confidence, contentment and satisfaction.

Adjustment involves the formation of an identity that integrates all aspects of the self, as well as an understanding at multiple levels of the meanings and implications disability has on the person's life. Major themes arising from such processes include: how individuals describe their difficulties; how they cope with specific limitations; and how they manage their identity and integrate their identity as a person with a disability into a cogent sense of self.

With specific reference to TBI, Simpson, Simons and McFadyen (2002) propose that the major challenge faced by people after TBI is reaching an understanding of exactly how the injury has affected their cognitive and psychosocial abilities. They experience an uncertainty about the full impact of the TBI throughout the period of recovery, rehabilitation and longer-term adjustment. The full impact of the injury may remain 'hidden' for some time.

TBI clients may be long-term patients and it is not unusual for them to be cared for within the hospital ward for up to two years. There are two distinct periods within the recovery period when clients are most vulnerable and confronting adjustment issues:

Stage 1 The first period usually occurs as they approach the stage of rehabilitation where progress begins to slow and there is a growing realization that a full recovery is becoming less likely.

Stage 2 The second period of vulnerability occurs between 6 to 12 months after discharge. On initial discharge, there is excitement about leaving the hospital and returning home. However, as this excitement wears off and the reality of long-term life changes is contemplated, boredom and depression may ensue.

Appropriately timing the inclusion of this method into therapy programmes with this population is crucial, and it is at these particular two phases of recovery from TBI where songwriting interventions can be especially valuable. Clinicians need to consider the appropriate timing in which to encourage reflection and adjustment through songwriting. The music therapist has an ethical duty to safeguard the emotional well-being of clients by not raising issues of which the client is not yet aware or emotionally ready to deal with. When client recovery is active, full participation in rehabilitation is essential. During this important phase of treatment, music therapists also need to make a clinical decision as to whether exploring adjustment issues are appropriate at that time. Reflecting and reviewing one's situation can lead to temporary crises when moments of insight occur and this may be detrimental to a client's treatment programme. More appropriate is the inclusion of self-reflection through songwriting when the client's rehabilitation is being hampered by negative emotional responses. In this situation, a client needs to work through these issues in order to maintain motivation for continued therapy.

Exploration through song

Coping and adjusting to trauma has been promoted within our therapy programmes by facilitating client exploration of thoughts, feelings and reactions to their acquired injury through songwriting. In analysing the lyrics of 82 songs written by clients with TBI, several themes emerged within the songs which could be directly related to aspects of patient adjustment to injury. These have been detailed in a number of our recent publications (Baker, Kennelly and Tamplin in press[a], in press[b], in press[c]). In particular, clients described feelings about, and responses towards, their present situation including the distress and pain involved in the hospitalization process and the feelings of isolation, dependency, helplessness and anger associated with their current situation. Many clients voiced concerns about how their physical and cognitive impairments caused others to view them, thus articulating confronting and painful issues related to body image (Charmaz 1995). Positive experiences were also included within songs, particularly experiences related to memories about, and reflections upon, significant others. When connecting with the positive aspects of

delay the process until the next session. It can also be useful for the client to take away some record of a song's progress at the end of a session. This may be in the form of a written copy of the song ideas and/or lyrics or a recording of the unfinished song so that he or she can prepare new ideas or changes between sessions.

Beginning a new song: lyric creation

The most common way to start writing a new song is to brainstorm ideas and record these on paper. This may often follow a period of discussion where the client is encouraged to talk about issues that are important or troubling and express their feelings about these issues. The client is then encouraged to select a topic or theme that has arisen out of this discussion from which ideas for lyrics may be generated. This process, entitled Therapeutic Lyric Creation (TLC), often follows a fairly standard format and has been developed over time by the authors:

Stage 1 Generate a range of topics to write about.

Stage 2 Select a topic for further exploration.

Stage 3 Brainstorm ideas directly related to the chosen topic.

Stage 4 Identify the principal idea/thought/emotion/concept within the topic (which functions as the focus of the chorus).

Stage 5 Develop the ideas identified as central to the topic.

Stage 6 Group related points together.

Stage 7 Discard the irrelevant or the least important points.

Stage 8 Construct an outline of the main themes within the song.

Stage 9 Construct the lyrics for the song.

In building client confidence with songwriting, it is often most appropriate to start with this general brainstorming of thoughts and ideas. This allows the flow of ideas to begin and expression is not impeded by the need for lyrical structure yet. In spite of a client's ability (or non-ability) to write, it is often best if the therapist scribes the ideas as this allows the client to talk freely and without interruption to the thought process. The therapist should take care to transcribe what the client says verbatim, so as to preserve the integrity and authenticity of the client's ideas. These ideas may be reworded or reorganized later on in the process to fit into a lyrical structure. The therapist should also provide the appropriate degree of support to facilitate the client's expression of ideas. This may consist of asking questions about statemer that the client has made or asking the client to expand on certain statements. It is also therapeutically important for the therapist to validate and encourage clients in their expression of significant personal issues. For clients who have difficulty with initiation, this initial process may be more productive if the therapist takes the role of an interviewer and asks the client key questions about issues which have been highlighted as being significant. For example, a client may make a statement such as 'I hate being in hospital', but have difficulty explicating why he or she hates it, or providing more information about his or her emotional responses. In this situation, the therapist may ask open-ended questions such as 'what is it, in particular, about being in hospital that you dislike?' or 'describe to me what it's like for you to be here'.

Fill-in-the-Blank and Song Parody Techniques

Alternatively, a Fill-in-the-Blank Technique (FBT) using a familiar song may be adopted. This technique has been previously described in the literature (Freed 1987; Goldstein 1990; Robb 1996). A song that the client relates to may be used and adapted to make it more personally relevant. For example, a song by Moving Pictures could be adapted and presented as follows:

> What about me? It isn't fair
> I've had enough
> Now get me out of here
> Can't you see? I want to be free
> But every day I'm stuck in here.

Here, clients complete the lyrics by including words or phrases that were brainstormed earlier in the process. This technique provides more structure for clients who may have difficulty expanding and organizing simple ideas. It can also provide direction for the lyrics and may serve as a beginning point for a client who is having trouble getting started.

Song Parody Technique (SPT) uses the music of a pre-composed song whereby the lyrics of the original song are completely replaced by client-generated lyrics. In many cases, a combination of these two techniques is employed.

In our clinical experience, SPT and FBT are the most commonly chosen and adopted methods with paediatric patients. Due to their developmental stage, many paediatric patients have not developed an individual music identity separate from their peers. Therefore, they are drawn to specific popular songs and musical artists. The very nature of this technique avoids the need for paediatric patients to make decisions about musical elements which may be too abstract for them at this developmental stage. This may be further compounded by impaired cognitive functioning as a result of a TBI.

Song Collage Technique

Another technique, which can be helpful for clients who have difficulty identifying or articulating their emotions, is the use of Song Collage Technique (SCT). This technique involves the client looking through music books or the lyric sheet within CD covers and selecting words or phrases from pre-composed songs that stand out, or have personal significance to them. The therapist facilitates this process by presenting a selection of songs which he/she considers contain meanings or descriptions of situations with which the client may resonate or identify. In these situations, identifying with the messages of other songs can enhance this therapeutic process. The clients can then add ideas to these words and phrases and reorganize or reword them into their own song lyrics.

The collection of words and phrases is similar to the brainstorming process mentioned earlier. In a similar way, like ideas are then grouped together and reordered to suit the client's preferences. The therapist encourages and supports the client in changing any necessary words, expanding ideas and adding phrases to link the different points within the song.

Use of Rhyme Technique

The use of rhyming lyric patterns herein termed the Use of Rhyme Technique (URT) can be employed to create structure in a song. The therapist should make a decision whether or not to introduce this option based on the client's cognitive abilities. If a client is able to generate lists of words that rhyme with key words which they have included, then this technique is a good way to expand and organize song ideas, for example sad/bad/mad/glad/dad.

If a client writes a song line such as 'being here just makes me sad', a list of words rhyming with sad (bad, mad, glad, dad, had) can be generated and one of these words that fits in with a previously brainstormed idea can be used, or the rhyming word can be used to generate a new idea. For example, 'being here just makes me sad, but I'll take the good with the bad', or 'being here just makes me sad, but I remember the good times that I've had'. Depending on the clients' cognitive abilities, the therapist may suggest phrases using the rhyming words that the clients have generated or the therapist may generate a list of rhyming words and ask the clients which word they relate to most and ask them to create the next phrase ending with this word.

Music composition

Often the music is created after at least some of the lyric creation has been completed. This is generally because many clients attending music therapy are not musicians themselves and feel most comfortable with the lyric creation part of the songwriting process. It is important to build the clients' confidence with a task with which they are more comfortable before introducing a more challenging or demanding task. The specialized skills of the music therapist are employed in explaining the music creation process and involving the clients in this process to the greatest degree possible. At the start of the songwriting process, clients are given the option of writing their own music, or using the music to a familiar song of their choice to which to write their own lyrics (SPT).

SPT is useful when clients feel daunted by the idea of writing music for their song, or when clients have difficulty conceptualizing how to structure a lyrical line without music. The use of pre-composed music can provide this sense of structure and gives the client guidelines for how many words or syllables for a line and how many lines for a verse or chorus. For some clients this sense of a familiar structure provides a feeling of security; however, for others it may be too limiting. It can sometimes be difficult to try to fit an idea for a lyrical line into the musical structure of a pre-composed song line. In some cases the integrity of clients' ideas may be better preserved if they do not have to change an idea in order to fit it into an existing rhythmic or melodic structure. Clients are then able to write lyrics freely and the music is composed to meld with the structure of the lyrics.

Musical genre and style

A good place to start the music creation is with the clients' preference for musical genre. This ground is familiar to most people, musicians and non-musicians alike. Most clients are able to state which genres of music they like or listen to, and if they cannot, the therapist can often determine this by asking the clients which artists or bands they like. It is important for the therapist to use language that the client can understand in order to promote maximum control and ownership of the music. It is often useful to ask questions about genre preference in relation to specific artists. For example, 'Do you want the music for your song to sound like a Metallica song or a Ben Harper song?'

Once the genre has been selected, different accompaniment styles can be presented for the client to choose between. These ideas may be improvised on an instrument by the therapist or trialled using an electronic keyboard accompaniment program or computer software. The choice of instrumentation is often determined by genre preference. For example, it is very difficult to create authentic sounding hip hop music using only an acoustic guitar. For this style of music, the use of computer software with recorded samples and loops and/or keyboards with pre-programmed accompaniments may be more appropriate. If a guitar is used, different accompaniment styles such as finger picking, pizzicato chords or strummed chords may be presented and different stylistic ideas, such as reggae or bossanova rhythmic patterns, power chords, standard blues riffs or use of a slide, offered as appropriate. Using a piano or electronic keyboard, arpeggios, octaves or chords may be presented as accompaniment options. The ideas for harmonic progressions are often best presented by the therapist as improvised passages, unless the client is musically proficient. Most clients will be able to identify aurally which harmonic progressions they like or think fit best with the feel of their song.

If the client is happy to sing in order to work out melody lines, then this is the next step in the song creation process. However, in our experience, even those clients who enjoy singing often don't feel confident or comfortable in using their voice to compose melody lines. The most common method we have found for melody composition is for the therapist to provide melody options for the client to listen to and choose between. The client is also encouraged to make independent decisions about the direction of the melody line; for example, 'Do you want the end of this line to go up or down?' Providing maximum opportunity for the client to contribute to the music composition ensures greater ownership of the completed song. Similar questions in terms of the range of dynamics and tempi to be used may also be asked to the client when completing the songwriting process.

Applications of the song post-recording

A recording and written transcription of the completed song is given to the client following completion of the lyrics and music. The song may be recorded on cassette tape, or for a better quality recording, a minidisc recording can be downloaded onto a computer and burnt onto a CD. These recordings serve as a record of the therapeutic songwriting process and can be used by clients to validate their emotional journey.

Some songs may be used:

- to communicate messages to loved ones
- to record positive past memories and experiences
- for self-motivation and encouragement during difficult times
- to affirm and encourage other clients who may be experiencing similar difficulties.

Sometimes when working with children, picture books including photos of children, their family, home and friends can also be incorporated with the final transcription of the song so as to provide a more visual/pictorial image of the song created.

Case example: A filthy song – genre to match emotional intensity

Sam was a young man aged 19 when he was referred for music therapy. He had received a severe traumatic brain injury resulting from a train accident. There was uncertainty surrounding the circumstances of the accident and whether it was an attempted suicide. Sam was very physically disabled as a result of his brain injury. His speech was severely dysarthric and consequently difficult to understand. His legs had both been broken in the accident, and he had high muscle tone resulting from the brain injury that caused him a lot of pain in physiotherapy. In addition to these physical issues, Sam also had severe cognitive and behavioural issues that affected his ability to participate in his rehabilitation. He was an angry young man, with limited insight into his disabilities and need for rehabilitation. Prior to music therapy intervention, his therapy sessions were often cancelled or ended prematurely due to non-compliance or aggression. As Sam's rehabilitation progress was being hindered by his negative emotional responses and behaviour, he was referred to music therapy for emotional expression and communication needs. The opportunity for self-reflection and expression through songwriting was considered appropriate as Sam needed to work through these issues in order to maintain motivation for continued therapy.

The songwriting process was not introduced into music therapy sessions until Sam had participated in music therapy for some time and rapport between the music therapist and Sam had been established. This foundation of trust and openness led Sam to feel comfortable talking with the music therapist about his feelings. This process of rapport building was further enhanced through making music with Sam which he enjoyed and to which he related. The music therapist introduced the concept of songwriting to Sam as a potential vehicle through which he could express and capture his emotional processes. Sam had a strong emotional connection to music and therefore he was responsive to this idea. He had a particular love of heavy metal music and this was the genre he wished to use for his song.

Sam's first song was written over three sessions, and evolved very much spontaneously rather than as a reorganization of the generated ideas. In brain storming, Sam's ideas were mostly phrases full of emotional intensity. Prior to his accident Sam was studying acting and his song lyrics reflected his artistic temperament. His ideas flowed quickly and remained largely unchanged in the final version of the song. As this song was very cathartic in nature, it was important to retain the ideas in their original form to capture the intensity of emotion expressed. This is the final version of his song lyrics. The name of the place where he lives has been omitted for confidentiality.

A filthy song

Chorus
I feel like shit, I hate it here
I miss my friends, wish they were near
I feel so bad, I want to walk again like I used to do
I love my dad because he believes in me.

Verse I
I hate this place it bores me to tears
And I feel like nothing in this universe
I hate this place I'm sick of it
Want to escape from this hell hole that I'm in
I want to go home…

Chorus

Verse 2
I was riding on a train one day
Going home to X where I've lived all my life
Both my legs were broken, they were hanging out the door
Of the train, then I passed out and I don't remember anything after that
Then I woke up here in hell.

Incorporating Sam's preference for heavy metal music and the intense negative emotions that he was expressing, a range of musical ideas and options for accompaniment style were presented for him to choose between. Sam selected minor chords to start both the verse and chorus as well as major–minor chord shifts (e.g. A major to A minor) at points within the song which may have reflected the intensity of sadness and anger he was experiencing. This contrast of emotions was also represented through a change in accompaniment style. The lyrics in the chorus expressed sadness and apathy and were represented musically through a melodic and sparse vocal line. The verses expressed anger and frustration and this was represented by a change in tonality, a more driving strumming style and an increase in dynamics. The melodic range was limited to four semitones and the use of a shifting C and C# creating musical tension and lack of change. A bridge of six bars between each verse and chorus was created using previously unused chords to express a new depth of emotion. In this part, the melody line finishes on the highest pitch within the song as if to emphasize the importance of this particular line.

This first song that Sam wrote in music therapy clearly expressed many emotional responses that he was experiencing, including loss, grief, anger, boredom and love. In it he also tells his story, the story of his accident, injury and hospitalization experience. The finished song was then recorded and the final version of the song is illustrated in Figure 6.1.

Sam wrote several songs in music therapy over the course of his inpatient rehabilitation programme. His second song explored fears of life after death and past antisocial drug-taking behaviour. The next song in his process focused on the physical pain and frustration of undertaking rehabilitation, specifically physiotherapy. It also addressed issues of body image. The final song written in his process addressed issues of the future, particularly going home and the desire for a relationship. Songwriting became a medium to document his adjustment process.

Sam's songs had other therapeutic applications in that he was able to listen to the recordings of the finished songs for self-motivation and validation of his emotions.

Case example: 'Wannabe' like a Spice Girl – song parody and musical identity

Sally was almost aged 12 when she was involved as a pedestrian in a motor vehicle accident where she sustained multiple traumas, including a severe head injury. As Sally progressed through PTA she received joint music therapy and speech pathology sessions which focused on two main areas: dysarthria and language difficulties. Her cognitive difficulties included memory impairment, psychomotor slowing, impaired problem-solving, rigid thinking and impaired social judgement. Sally was unmotivated to participate in most therapy sessions. Therefore a referral for individual music therapy sessions was made to address her emotional needs including self-expression and adjustment to hospitalization.

Music therapy assessment revealed that Sally enjoyed listening to and playing music. She had previously learnt the piano and the clarinet at school and enjoyed listening to a variety of age-appropriate popular music, particularly the Spice Girls. To address the need for self-expression, songwriting was offered to Sally and she chose to use song parody as her preferred method. She was excited about the idea of producing her own songs and chose to use the music of a popular Spice Girls song 'Wannabe' to which to write her own lyrics. This demonstrates that song parody, in particular the use of current popular songs, is the preferred method of songwriting with this age group.

Sally appeared to have little difficulty in creating ideas for lyrics, but her dysarthria adversely affected her ability to articulate her intended speech

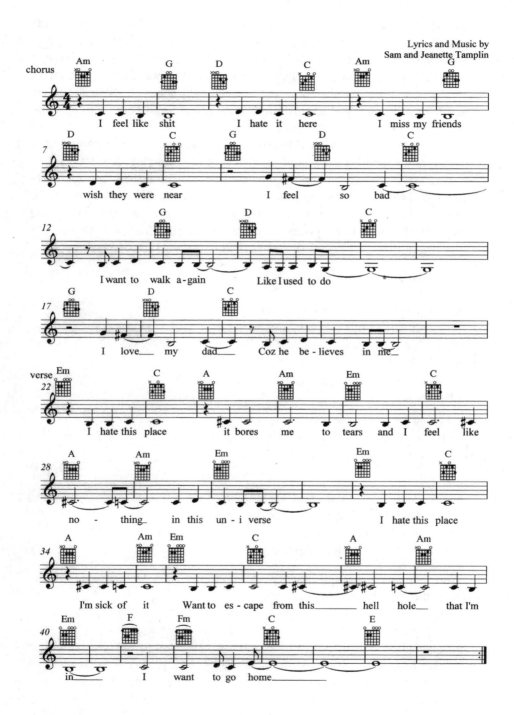

Figure 6.1 Final version of 'A filthy song'

clearly. Sally's mother was more familiar with Sally's way of speaking and was present for most sessions. Her mother was able to assist Sally if she was experiencing difficulties in articulating her thoughts and ideas. Based on clinical experience with this population, the music therapist offered Sally a selection of subject choices for her song – family, home and hospital. Sally chose to write about her experiences in hospital, which included relationships with staff members and descriptions of negative aspects of her hospital experience.

The use of song parody provided the necessary structure and predictability of melody and rhythm to aid the organization of her ideas into a lyrical format. Sally was always quick to remind the music therapist if her lyrics were not interpreted accurately. Sally was often excited during this songwriting process and often wanted to perform actions to the songs while in her wheelchair. During these times she would often need to be reminded to remain focused on the songwriting activity. These are the lyrics to the final version of Sally's song.

Naughty nurses
Verse 1
I'll tell you what I want what I really really want
I want to get out of this dumb stupid hospital
I hate medicine medicine makes me feel sicker
Except for Baclofen

Chorus
If you want to be so naughty you've got to be like Tracey
Tracey is my favourite and she is the best
Christine and Rebecca, they're my favourites too
But hospital is so smelly 'cause I think it is

Verse 2
I'll tell you what I like what I really really like
I like Sam because she does OT with me
and then there's Prue 'cause I just like her
There's no real reason I just like her

She was promised an opportunity to videotape her performance of the completed song with actions included.

Before Sally was discharged she expressed a need to write a 'going home' song. During these final therapy sessions she would often speak of being excited about leaving hospital and because this date was so close to Christmas and her twelfth birthday, there were so many family events, holiday activities and of course presents to which to look forward. This resulted in another song parody being created using yet another Spice Girls song, 'Stop Right Now'. This song spoke of her family members, events to which she was looking forward and also the desire to walk again. Both of these song parodies were video-recorded and presented in booklet form together with pictures of Sally and her family which she was then able to take home and share with family and friends.

While these were the only two songs that Sally wrote during her rehabilitation, each song parody described two significant moments in her life – her own experience of being in hospital and also preparations for the future and returning home. Song parody provided Sally with the opportunity to express a variety of emotions, thoughts and feelings which not only assisted her adjustment to hospital but also to her future as she returned home to begin a new life.

Conclusions

This chapter has primarily addressed the therapeutic rationale for introducing songwriting to TBI clients. Songwriting can facilitate the expression of emotions and assist in the movement towards emotional adjustment. Some of the more relevant and effective therapeutic techniques used when writing songs with TBI clients have been outlined. In particular, techniques such as song parody, fill-in-the-blank, song collage and the use of rhyme can be appropriate strategies to manage the cognitive deficits with which these clients may present. At the same time these techniques can be used to encourage the creation of lyrics which express feelings. In writing song lyrics, clients have opportunities to explore their own reactions to the issues addressed within the song. This is a vital step in coming to terms with the trauma that they have experienced and the short- and long-term implications of this trauma that have so adversely impacted upon their lives.

The chapter has also highlighted the importance of creating genres of music that are appealing to the client. We have particularly emphasized the attention to detail in the selection of the accompaniment style for a client's song. The use of samples, loops and pre-programmed accompaniment styles within music software programs and modern electric keyboards can be used effectively to create genre-specific effects. When using guitar accompaniment, it is important to talk with the client about how they want the song to sound and experiment with different guitar strumming and picking styles (bossanova, reggae, ballad, hard rock, etc.) to create the feel and genre for the song that is desired.

Music therapists working in rehabilitation must be flexible, creative and adaptive in their therapeutic approach to songwriting. The techniques presented in this chapter need to be at the fingertips of the informed therapist in order to facilitate clear clinical decision-making about the method of presentation. This, in turn, offers maximum choice and control over the song creation process to the TBI client, in a manner appropriate to their level of need.

7

Working with Impairments in Pragmatics through Songwriting following Traumatic Brain Injury

Felicity Baker

Songwriting for and with patients who have Traumatic Brain Injury (TBI) is an effective intervention for addressing a range of emotional, cognitive and communication impairments. Chapter 6 by Baker, Kennelly and Tamplin illustrated how the intervention can be applied to facilitate the process of adjustment being faced by patients who have experienced brain trauma. This chapter examines the more functional use of songwriting with this population where the intervention is specifically applied to address acquired impairments in pragmatics. The chapter first outlines the pragmatic skills necessary to create appropriate conversations and describes the typical presentation of pragmatic impairments often present in people with TBI. Following this, I explain my views on why songwriting is suitable for addressing impairments in pragmatics by illustrating the similarities between how conversations and songs are constructed. The procedures for implementing the songwriting intervention are then outlined and two vignettes exemplify these procedures.

Pragmatic disorders

While only a minority of TBI patients suffer clinical aphasic syndromes where speech and language are severely impaired, a significant proportion of patients with TBI experience long-term problems with their communication abilities and consequently jeopardize their potential to develop and maintain meaningful relationships with others (Biddle, McCabe and Bliss 1996; Kasher *et al.* 1999). Evidence suggests that these patients, while able to use basic linguistic processes normally, frequently have difficulty adapting their communication productions to meet the specific needs of the context. Such patients may be described as over-talkative and tangential, or under-talkative, as having inadequate specificity, impaired turn-taking, or poor topic maintenance. Patients fitting this description are said to be presenting with impairments in pragmatics. 'Language pragmatics' is the term used to describe the application of language and behaviour to convey meaning (Adams 2002). Therefore, the term 'pragmatic disorder' describes the mismatch between language and the context in which it was used.

An analysis and classification of the difficulties in pragmatic competency was first described by Grice (1978). He developed a model of conversational practice, which has since been adopted to clinically assess patients with pragmatic disorders (Adams 2002; Borod *et al.* 2000; Kasher *et al.* 1999). Grice (1978) proposed that appropriate conversations contained the following:

1. *Specificity* – The discourse conveys specific, unambiguous information.

2. *Topic maintenance* – A series of utterances share a theme and a topic is maintained and developed.

3. *Relevancy* – The selection of topics relate to the matter under consideration. All remarks are relevant.

4. *Conciseness* – The utterances are informative but not too informative. There are no unnecessary details.

5. *Quantity* – The content of the utterance is complete.

6. *Lexical selection* – The selection of words and sentences fit the text. There is no evidence of word-finding difficulties and there is an appropriate and wide selection of words.

Many patients with TBI present with substantial impairments in pragmatic competency. They may provide too much or too little information, or much of the information supplied by them is superfluous or was not requested of them. Some of the content of their conversations may be inaccurate or at times blatantly false, or their conversation may contain contradictory statements. In communicating with others, their statements may bear no relevance or relation to previous statements and they may have impairments in the development and maintenance of topics. For example, they may have difficulty introducing or continuing with a topic, and they may frequently shift to unrelated topics (topic shift) or topics that are linked together (topic chain). Further, patients may reuse previous topics (topic recycling and topic reintroduction), and are unable to initiate and develop conversations based on more than a couple of familiar topics (Adams 2002). Overcoming problems with pragmatics depends on patients being aware of these impairments and an intact ability to monitor their own conversations ensuring that they are appropriate to the context. Perhaps the greatest factor limiting progress in patients with TBI is their impairment in these higher order cognitive skills. Therefore clinicians considering addressing impairments of pragmatic disorders need to consider addressing the issues of self-awareness, self-monitoring, impulse control and perseveration.

Songs as mirrors of conversational skills

The creation of song lyrics is akin to the process of creating conversations and can therefore be considered a suitable medium for redeveloping conversational skills in people with TBI. For example, in creating lyrics, the songwriter must first choose a topic or focus for the song (be it fact or fiction). Once the topic has been decided upon, he then explores and describes the different aspects of that topic, using language statements accurately to portray its dimensions. Once these statements have been collated, the songwriter considers which points are most salient and call for emphasis within the song. In these cases, these statements are often adapted to shape the chorus of a song. The remaining points are then reviewed. Some may be discarded if no longer considered relevant, and others may be reordered, further explored and developed, and then adapted to form the verses to support the chorus.

Given the parallels between the process of creating lyrics and creating conversations, songwriting lends itself beautifully to being a tool to address pragmatic disorders in people with TBI. Songs can be created around an unlimited number of factual or fictional topics that might not be otherwise easy to 'practise' in general conversation. Patients can create songs around personal information such as self-reflections, relationships with significant others, leisure interests, past, present or future events and even day-to-day topics such as the weather. In doing this, they develop a repertoire of topics which they can confidently use when talking to others, and also develop a set of strategies to assist them in participating in discussions with others. Patients learn not just to initiate a range of topics, but to develop them, have an opinion about them, and create conversational turn-taking opportunities with others using a series of open rather than closed statements.

Setting goals and introducing songwriting as an intervention

Within my protocol of treatment, in almost all cases, patients are introduced to the idea of writing songs as soon as I have identified that pragmatic skill redevelopment is a priority area for their rehabilitation.[1] Identification of pragmatic impairments may have arisen through meeting the patient in the first session and talking with him or her, or through referral from the speech and language therapist. In my experience I have never found it appropriate to commence songwriting during the first meeting with a patient; there have, however, been numerous occasions where this was appropriate during the second session.

The concept of songwriting is introduced and explained to patients as being a task which can help them to be more proficient when conversing with others. In some instances, patients experience anxiety about their ability to create songs and therefore reinforcing the support that the therapist will offer them is imperative from the beginning. When patients are overly anxious about all aspects of their therapy treatment, I will often introduce the concept of songwriting by playing and singing them a song written by another patient.[2]

Prior to therapy commencing, goals are set and agreed upon between patient and therapist. Within neurorehabilitation programmes in Australia, the inter-disciplinary team demand that goals be concrete, functional and, in most cases, clearly observable before approval for providing services will be given.[3] Examples of goals with a patient might be as follows:

- To work on generating three new and related ideas (for insertion into a song) with minimum prompting.

- To correctly identify and discard the two least relevant points from the list of points generated about a topic.

---

1   Patients may have clear difficulties with pragmatics; however, these will not be directly addressed within my therapy programme if they present with other impairments that are deemed by the treatment team as higher priorities.

2   In these cases, I have always asked for permission from the client to play his/her songs to other clients; this in itself has therapeutic value for the songwriter.

3   Some music therapists might argue that these goals are too limiting for therapy in that creativity and spontaneity is sacrificed in order to meet these goals. However, in my opinion creativity and spontaneity are actually encouraged by encouraging the patients to extend their skills – resulting in a greater potential for accurate self-expression in daily living.

·onsistently self-monitor the length (quantity) of his contributions
᠆uring the creation of song lyrics).

Once appropriate goals are in place, the therapy sessions can commence.

Creation of lyrics

When patients with TBI write songs, the lyrics are usually created first. This principle has evolved after witnessing the frustration that some patients experience when they are unable to create lyrics that fit into the previously determined structure of the music. Additionally, creating lyrics (words) is more concrete and familiar than creating music, and given the cognitive difficulties in processing abstract information which is typical of this population, I have found that creating the lyrics prior to the music has been the most consistently successful approach when working with this population and forms a fairly consistent format. This approach, which I describe as Therapeutic Lyric Creation (TLC), has been developed and refined through my work over the past 12 years and through the influential writings of O'Callaghan (1996) in her work with palliative care patients. The main stages within my approach, as seen in Chapter 6, are:

Stage 1 Generate a range of topics to write about.

Stage 2 Select a topic for further exploration.

Stage 3 Brainstorm ideas directly related to the chosen topic.

Stage 4 Identify the principal idea/thought/emotion/concept within the topic (which functions as the focus of the chorus).

Stage 5 Develop the ideas identified as central to the topic.

Stage 6 Group related points together.

Stage 7 Discard the irrelevant or the least important points.

Stage 8 Construct an outline of the main themes within the song.

Stage 9 Construct the lyrics for the song.

Throughout this process, feedback and strategies are provided by the therapist to facilitate the songwriting process and to provide sufficient structure to enable the patients to become more independent and better able to participate in and develop interesting conversations with others.

Stage 1: generating a range of topics to write about

When asked to choose a topic about which to write a song, patients may tell you that they have no idea about what to choose and often cannot offer even a single idea. On most occasions, this is an impulsive response, and the patient has not attempted to think of a topic. When this occurs, the therapist can encourage the patient to think more carefully. In some instances, at the beginning of the patient's therapy programme, the therapist may provide him or her with possible options. Typical examples of suggested topics might be: family, hospital, holidays, leisure activities, work/school, hospital staff, etc.

Stage 2: selection of a topic for further exploration

The patients are then encouraged to make a choice about what they would like to write about. It is often necessary to support patients in making these choices by encouraging them to think about what interests them the most, what is the most important topic to them at this present moment, what they would like to talk about most, and what they might like to share with other patients/staff/family/friends.

Stage 3: brainstorm ideas directly related to the chosen topic

In developing the topic, patients are often challenged by the 'limits' placed upon them by the exercise. They are encouraged to remain 'on topic'. When patients provide inappropriate, irrelevant and/or superfluous material, the therapist should offer the patient feedback about this. Patients who are significantly impaired or in the early stages of addressing pragmatics should receive feedback immediately. They need to be directly informed of what is inappropriate, irrelevant and/or superfluous, and why. As patients progress through therapy, and for the more high-functioning patients, the therapist should encourage them to reflect on their contributions and to self-monitor what was inappropriate or irrelevant in what they have said and why. At the same time, they are called on to justify why their ideas are important for the song. This is an essential step in their development of self-monitoring and self-awareness. Independence is promoted in the higher-functioning patients by providing them with set 'homework' tasks. Here, patients are provided with tasks such as to write down five points about *a given topic* which could be used to write a song about *the given topic*. It is expected that patients will return to therapy having completed these tasks where their work is then reviewed together with the therapist.

Stage 4: identify the principal idea/thought/emotion/concept within the topic

The patient and therapist then discuss the ideas and the patient is encouraged to identify which of the points raised within the brainstorming exercise are the most important to the patient and central to the theme of the song. This can either be factual (that is, there is truth or falsity to what they decide is most important) or it can be their view of what is the most important aspect of the topic. From these decisions, the principal theme of the song is decided upon and often material from this stage is used to construct a chorus. Patients may require some prompting and support to encourage them to make decisions about the key theme of the song. In brainstorming ideas during stage 3, often the central theme changes from the initial topic decided in stage 2 and this becomes most evident during stage 4 when the central theme is identified.

The patient is then encouraged to construct lyrics to form a chorus based on this central theme. The support provided by the therapist is dependent upon the abilities of the patient at that time. Suggested lyrics or key words might be offered, or the patient may be expected to construct the lyrics independently. In all cases, the patient is encouraged to extend his/her current skill level rather than be supported too intensely by the therapist.

Stage 5: develop the ideas identified as central to the topic

An important strategy that the therapist can utilize to assist patients in developing ideas for the song is to encourage them to use the 'wh' questions – what, which, where, when, why, who and how. These questions can be asked of many topics to expand and extrapolate the dimensions of the topic. If a patient wants to write a song about his favourite take-away food, say McDonald's (believe me, these are the types of topics patients want to write about sometimes!), then he could ask himself the questions:

What? What type of McDonald's food selections do I prefer – e.g. Big Mac, French Fries, Thickshakes?

Why? Why do I like McDonald's – e.g. image, taste, convenience?

Where? Where is the McDonald's that I visit the most – in town, near work?

When? When do I usually go to McDonald's – for breakfast, lunch or dinner, before/after a movie, etc. (and why)?

Who? With whom do I go to McDonald's – by myself, with family, friends, football team (and why)?

By asking patients to question themselves (or others if engaged in a conversation), they are able to form an opinion – they are not limited by a single idea of liking McDonald's food, but are able to express why they like it and develop something more specific to say about the issue.

Stage 6: group related points together

When the patient has saturated a topic, a key task within the songwriting process is the ability to group 'like' ideas together. These ideas which have a common theme form the basis of the verses. The patients are encouraged to consider carefully and be critical as to how and to what degree these ideas are related. This ability to self-monitor and be critical of their contributions is an important skill and essential for appropriate discourse.

Stage 7: discard the irrelevant or the least important points

During stage 6, patients often find one or more brainstormed ideas do not relate to other sub-themes. The patient and therapist can engage in conversations about whether these points are directly relevant or important to the song's central theme. Decisions at this point can be made to discard irrelevant or least important concepts. If the patient communicates that some of his/her points are necessary points for inclusion within the song, stage 5 can be revisited whereby these points are further elaborated and developed so there is sufficient detail to construct a verse around that sub-theme.

Stage 8: construct an outline of the main themes within the song

The final stage before creating the lyrics is to prepare an outline of the song whereby the sub-themes are ordered and reordered to provide a logical flow of ideas. From here, the points within each sub-theme are then ordered again so the ideas flow and make sense to the listener. This step is often difficult for patients with pragmatic impairments but a necessary skill for them to redevelop so that their conversations with others will also flow in a logical and understandable manner. The therapist encourages the patients to consider each sub-theme and points within the sub-theme and their relationship to other points as a starting point. Extending this idea, the therapist then encourages the patients critically to reflect and monitor their own work.

Stage 9: construct the lyrics for the song

The next task involved in songwriting is to create the actual lyrics. Patients are encouraged to select phrases from the previously grouped ideas and modify these to form lyrics that will fit into a phrase structure. They are asked to consider their selection of words. They are continuously questioned and challenged. 'Is this really what you are trying to say?' 'Is there another word that could describe your thoughts (or feelings/experiences/situations, etc.) more accurately?' 'Can you communicate the same idea in a more concise way so that it matches the length of the other song phrases?' After the lyrics have been written, the therapist and patient review the lyrics and make any necessary changes to ensure that the words accurately portray the communicative intentions of the patient, and to check that the phrases are relatively consistent in structure, length and metre. This consistency aids the music creation process.

The use of alternative modes of communication

Many patients with TBI are unable to communicate verbally and consequently utilize a range of alternative modes of communication. Some point to alphabet boards, or use eye-blinking/head nodding/shaking to indicate choices (on an alphabet board or picture board), other patients use electronic devices such as electronic talkers to communicate their messages. Patients might also employ makaton or sign language as their primary means of communication. Clinicians need to be aware that when writing songs with patients who use these alternative modes, the process is extremely slow as it may take them a long time to spell out simple statements. For example, it is not uncommon for these patients to take 30 minutes to spell out two sentences on an alphabet board. Frequently, patients would tire and forget half-way through a sentence what they were trying to say. This can be frustrating for the patient and clinicians need to keep the patient's motivation and satisfaction with the process in check. Structuring the song so that the lyrics can be short in length and allow for the possibility of repetition is one means of reducing the effects of fatigue while ensuring a musically and lyrically desirable effect. It is important for clinicians to remember that some of the best popular songs are built on repetition.

Contraindications arise when the patients' alternative modes of communication are limiting and do not allow him or her to express his or her thoughts precisely. In this situation, it is sometimes possible for the therapist to offer various elaborations on ideas and the patient is offered the opportunity to choose one that might align with his or her thinking.

Constructing the music

When constructing the music to accompany the lyrics, clinicians can select one of three general procedures: selection of genre first, construction of melody first or song parody. Their choice is dependent upon each specific patient or context.

Genre first

Patients that I treated at the rehabilitation hospital were often within the 18–35-year-old age group, and mostly males. This specific population has a strong connection with music and they tend to have clear ideas as to what style or genre of music they prefer. When this is the case, the genre guides the construction of the music.

Fortunately, modern electronic keyboards tend to have a multitude of in-built accompaniment styles which create the 'whole band' effect with drum rhythm, rhythmic guitar and keyboard arrangements – a wonderful tool for clinicians writing songs with patients. A range of styles from rhythm and blues, heavy metal, hip hop and Euro-pop (these being the most popular with my patient group) can be presented to patients where they can select a style of music that they like. The song can then be moulded around this in-built 'band'.

The next step in the process is to create a suitable harmonic progression. The therapist, continuing to have the accompaniment style sounding, improvises around different chord progressions, and asks the patients to signal when they like a certain 'effect'. Given the significant cognitive impairments evident within these patients, and their difficulties with abstract ideas, they are often drawn to predictable progressions. For those therapists/students who are most comfortable improvising around the key of C major and its relative key modulations (as I am), I have often used the harmonic progressions listed in Table 7.1 (in various combinations) as these predictable progressions tend to be the most popular with this population and suitable for their preferred genre of songs. You can of course modulate these to whatever key fits the melodic line of the song. In this table, each cell represents one bar of a four-beat measure (common time). The timing can be altered to suit the style of the song and the melody line of lyrics.

Table 7.1 Harmonic progressions useful in constructing songs

Bar 1	Bar 2	Bar 3	Bar 4
C maj	A min	D min	G maj
C maj	E min	F maj	G maj
C maj	D min	G maj	C maj
F maj	F min	C maj	C maj
E min	E min	F maj	F maj
D min	D min	G maj	G maj
E min	E min	A min	A min
D min	G maj	C maj	C maj
A♭ maj	A♭ maj	E♭ maj	E♭ maj
F min	F min	G maj	G maj
A♭ maj	A♭ maj	E♭ maj	E♭ maj
F maj	F maj	B♭ maj	B♭ maj
E♭ maj	E♭ maj	F min	F min
G maj	G maj	C min	C min
F min	F min	G maj	G maj

When they have identified a harmonic progression that is appealing to them, the therapist will often repeat this progression several times (again with the keyboard's in-built accompaniment style sounding) and improvise sung melodies over the top of this so that the lyrics fit into the standard four-bar phrase structure. Here, I try to create a 'catchy' and predictable melody line, ensuring that it suits the genre of the song. Clinicians need to be familiar with a variety of song genres when working with this population and be comfortable at improvising in these different styles. This will aid the music creation process. It is important to create melodies with a restricted vocal range (I suggest a maximum of an octave) that contain a limited number of intervals which are larger than a major third and include many major and minor second intervals. Further, the melody should be set at a medium register. These are important considerations as it is likely that the patients may want to sing and record their songs, and to do so the melodies need to be simple enough so as to be sung by non-musically trained people.

During this process, patients are asked to signal when a particular melody line is appealing. Sometimes patients are asked for their own suggestions and contributions. Choices about who makes the suggestions are dependent on the patient's initiative, communication abilities and the time available for writing the song. When patients are so physically impaired that they are unable to sing (or improvise melodies on a keyboard), they will be offered a range of different melodies from which to choose. Similarly, when songs need to be completed within a certain time frame because the patient is being discharged, the songwriting process is accelerated by introducing melodies from which the patient can choose.

Following the completion of the song, it should then be reviewed by both therapist and patient and small changes made to the melody line and tempo and sometimes lyrics might be altered slightly to increase the overall musical result. Instrumental 'fills' (again often in-built into keyboard programs), or changes in accompaniment style between the verses and chorus, can be added at this point to create a professional effect. Patients are usually impressed by the finished product.

Due to time constraints of working within the hospital, I rarely had sufficient time to notate the melody line. I usually made an audio-recording of each song to safeguard the integrity of the song's melody. Patients were often provided with a copy of this audio-recording for their own record of the therapy process.

Melody first

While choosing a genre was the more popular means of creating a song, in some cases the exact opposite procedure was employed. Here, several differing melodies are improvised by the therapist and the patients are asked to choose which melody line they prefer. Again it is important to consider creating melodies that are predictable and 'catchy' as well as being simple enough to be able to be sung by the patients themselves. In the higher-functioning patients, or where time allowed, the patients should be encouraged to create their own melodic line. In these cases, the therapist offers suggestions about how to refine or develop the melody. This might involve:

- changing the rhythm of the melody so that the lyrics flow better with the melody

- suggesting interval changes so the lyrics are more simple to sing

- suggesting repetition so that songs are more unified and more easily recalled.

Following the creation of the melody, different chord progressions, and later an accompaniment style (genre), are presented to the patients for their selection. This protocol is being adopted when patients are unable to identify a genre of music to which they would like to set their song.

Song parody

Due to the significant physical and cognitive impairments of some patients, song parody is often employed. Here, the original melody, harmony and genre of a known song is retained (or sometimes also varied), and new lyrics are created. This technique is valuable for patients with traumatic brain injury in that it provides them with a predetermined concrete structure through which to write their songs. Often it is more motivating than creating original songs as they can choose their favourite songs to re-write. With this technique, the therapist provides the link between the song and the patient's lyrics, musically demonstrating to the patient how their lyrics might fit within the songs and preserving the song's musical integrity.

The afterlife of the song

Once the song has been completed, it takes on a new life and purpose. An audio-recording and a transcribed version of the song (lyrics only) is given to the patient as a record. For longer-term patients, they are provided with a folder (termed 'song-folio', Lee and Baker 1997) where they keep a record of the songs they have written and this doubles as a record of their progress in therapy. They can review how the length of the songs has increased and how their language usage has improved over time. Further, the songs (and folios) also serve as 'topics of conversation' within themselves as patients can talk with others about the songs they have written, about why they selected each topic, and the process of writing the song. Here, they are practising their 'pragmatic skills' in out-of-therapy contexts.

Case example: Euro-pop, Boy Bands and boys

At the time I was working with Mary, she was a delightful 16-year-old girl who had received a severe TBI after being involved in a road traffic accident. Following her recovery from coma and post-traumatic amnesia, she was left with residual impairments in pragmatics. On assessment she was unable to initiate any conversation, thereby displaying significant pragmatic impairments in specificity, topic maintenance, relevancy, conciseness, quantity and lexical selection. She occasionally used short functional sentences but she usually responded to conversation with one of a small selection of phrases – 'ah-ha', 'yep', 'mmm', 'no', 'I don't know' and 'when's mum coming?' Crucial to her recovery was a need to develop her ability to converse with others. She was referred to music therapy for a number of reasons including the need to address her severe lack of initiation and conversational participation.

When I commenced therapy with Mary, she was not able independently to generate a song-topic. When I asked her to think of possible topics she sat there blankly looking at me and then responded with an 'I don't know'. Her impairments were so significant that I decided to complete the first stage of the songwriting process myself and move to the second stage by offering her a range of possible topics. Fortunately, I was familiar with Mary's interests and I knew she liked 'Boy Bands' and 'boys'. I included 'boys' within the topics I offered her, to which she immediately responded with excitement.

Before commencing the songwriting intervention, I discussed with Mary my thoughts about the focus of her therapy and Mary agreed that her therapy goal would be to develop at least five discussion points about boys which she could confidently discuss in conversations with her friends.

Over the course of three 40-minute sessions, I helped Mary to generate her ideas about what she liked and disliked about boys (stages 3 and 4 in the lyric creation process). By using the 'wh' questions described earlier, she was able to generate some key descriptive words. I then encouraged her to develop her ideas further (stage 5) by using these keywords as departure points and applying the 'wh' questions again to achieve this. For example, one such point she mentioned was that they needed to 'be good looking'. I encouraged her to be more specific by offering cues such as 'what does it mean to you to be good looking?', 'What colour eyes do you like?' and 'What type of body shape do you prefer?' Sometimes her ability to communicate her opinion was aided by offering her choices of responses. For example, I would ask her 'What style of boy do you like – should he be clean-cut, rough and ragged, sporty, surfer, skateboarder, rapper, etc?' In using the 'wh' questions, not only was she being encouraged to think and form an opinion, but I was helping her to create a repertoire of ideas on which she could draw when discussing 'boys' with her girlfriends.

The resulting large list of brainstormed and expanded ideas then needed to be grouped into related points (stage 6). Mary found this task difficult and maximum prompting was needed for her to link *like* ideas. Mary was able to communicate to me that a good body shape, good looks, eye colour and skin colour were the most important points she wanted to emphasize, so these were grouped together and later became the chorus. Following this, all points that were not able to be grouped together, or were not considered the most important points to Mary, were discarded (stage 7).

The final task in creating the lyrics for the song was actually to construct the lyrics of each verse and chorus. Mary was not able to initiate specific lyrics so I offered suggestions for lyrics and awaited her appraisal of my suggestions. Wherever possible I included Mary's own words – hence the song title 'Fish in the sea'. This is the final version of her lyrics:

Fish in the sea
Verse 1
So many fish in the sea out there
So many men but what do I care
Meeting nice men makes me feel good
Oh well, at least it should

Chorus
A muscle pack of six or four
Makes me wanna come back for more
Looking good but not rough and tough
Blue eyes, brown skin and all that stuff

Verse 2
They go crazy when they buy me flowers
At nightclubs they entertain me for hours
A bite to eat or a movie or two
Saying I'm beautiful will get them through

Chorus

Verse 3
He must dress well but no collar and tie
Otherwise I'll say good bye
If he has money I'd prefer a car
That would make him a real star

Chorus

In moving to the music creation, I asked Mary to nominate a style of music for the song to which she adopted a standard response – 'I don't know'. As Mary was a big fan of Boy Bands, I suggested to her that the song could be set to a Boy Band style music – something in the lines of Euro-pop. So in taking the 'genre first' approach, I provided examples of different Euro-pop styles by playing various pre-set accompaniment styles built into the keyboard and she was able to select one that appealed to her. The harmonic progression was then developed by improvising chord changes over the top of the accompaniment until Mary had identified the progressions that appealed to her the most.

From there, melody lines were improvised until Mary identified the ones she liked. Care was taken to ensure that the melody line was simple and easily able to be sung. At that time, some of the lyrics were then modified so as to maintain the style of the song but still bring across Mary's intended message. A

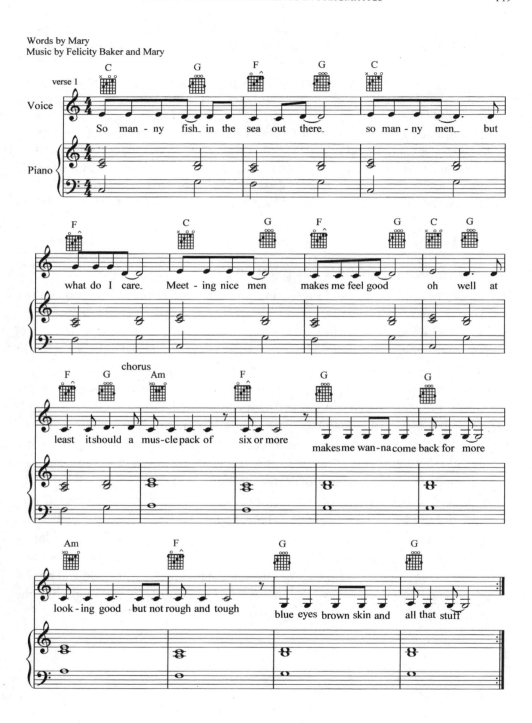

Figure 7.1 Final version of 'Fish in the sea'

variation in the accompaniment style was added and separated by an instrumental fill to differentiate the chorus from the verse. Figure 7.1 illustrates the
final version.

In Mary's case, creating a song about boys gave her an opportunity to
become aware of a range of thoughts and opinions about boys, which she could
share with her school friends when they came to visit her in hospital. She
became able to articulate specific likes and dislikes, these being age appropriate
and engaging for her peers. Participation in therapeutic lyric creation continued
within her music therapy programme and she created additional songs. As an
outcome, Mary began to cease saying 'I don't know' and instead began to initiate
and engage in conversations as an active participant rather than a passive
listener only.

Assessing skills through songwriting

An important function of the songwriting process is that it provides opportunities
for assessment of a patient's therapy progress. A patient's performance can be
compared with previous performances within sessions and compared with the performances of other patients. Table 7.2 illustrates a simple method a therapist might
employ in creating an overall picture of a patient's level of pragmatic functioning. It
is important when recording the assessment that the therapist provides sufficient
detail about the level of prompting and support required by the patient (independent, minimal, moderate, maximum prompting) so that an accurate picture of the
patient's level of independence is recorded.

In the example below, I have used the case example of Craig to illustrate how
this assessment format can be applied. Here, it can be seen that Craig mostly contributed an appropriate amount of information, and that his information was always
accurate (I don't know much about Ford cars so I had to trust him!) and consistent.
Craig had difficulty maintaining topic and his statements were not always closely
related to the direction of the conversation. Craig was not perseverative and
therefore did not repeat or reintroduce information previously discussed and he was
mostly good at being able to expand his ideas with little prompting from the
therapist.

Table 7.2 Assessment of Craig's therapy participation in session 3

Skills evaluated	Never	Sometimes	Mostly	Always
Quantity of information is appropriate			✓	
Information is accurate				✓
Information is consistent (i.e. no contradictory statements)				✓
Information is relevant to and links with preceding statements		✓		
Topic is maintained		✓		
Information is not repeated (recycled/reintroduced topics/points)				✓
Topic is developed			✓	
Ideas are ordered into related groups	N/A			
Least relevant ideas are discarded	N/A			
Patient self-corrects inappropriate, irrelevant, repeated information		✓		
Contributes ideas non-impulsively		✓		
Does not perseverate on same idea/topic		✓		
Does not perseverate on same sentence/sentence structure	✓			
Uses large range of adjectives and adverbs to describe details			✓	

Case example: Ford cars and Guns 'n' Roses

Daniel and Craig were two young men in their early to mid-30s and had been in hospital for more than a year at the time they were being seen for individual music therapy. Both men shared the same hospital room and displayed similar impairments in that they were both non-verbal, used alphabet boards to communicate, and were both substantially impaired in their conversational skills. Due to Daniel and Craig's severe TBI, they also fatigued easily and communication with them was slow. Both also had a terrific sense of humour. As they shared a room, hospital staff attempted to encourage interaction between them, but this was difficult due to the severe level of communication problems evident in both of them. It was decided to trial a joint music therapy session with the two patients with the view that the conversational practice emerging within the sessions might lead to the development of a meaningful co-patient relationship.

Having worked with both of these patients before, I knew their interests well, and knowing their rapid developing fatigue, I decided to offer them suggestions for topics rather than using the therapy time for them to come up with their own ideas. The suggestions I gave them were cars, music, parties and women. They were also offered the possibility of generating a completely different topic if they had the desire to do so. Cars – Ford Falcons to be specific – were the obvious choice as far as they were concerned.

At this point I offered them two possibilities – to create a completely original song or to change the lyrics of a well-known song (song parody). They decided that they would like to change the lyrics to the Guns 'n' Roses song 'Sweet child of mine' and called their new song 'Sweet Ford of mine'.

The next three therapy sessions were spent brainstorming points to be included in the song (step 3). This was a time-consuming process as they were very slow at pointing to the alphabet board and often became distracted. The 'wh' questions were used to draw out their ideas and thoughts about cars; for example, 'What makes a Ford Falcon such a good car?', 'What model is the best Falcon?'

Craig and Daniel had a lot of fun in grouping related ideas together (step 6) and did not discard any of the ideas they had initiated (step 7) as they argued that anything to do with Fords was important. I constructed the lyrics of the song using some of the same words offered by Craig and Daniel. As neither of these patients could vocalize or sing, I made a recording of the song for them. They both laugh every time they play the song as they find it amusing and it has become not only a conversational point between each other and their families and friends, but it was also the instigator in the development of a friendship between these two patients. These are the final lyrics of the song ('carbie', in verse 2, is slang for carburettor):

Sweet Ford of mine
Verse 1
The best car in the world is the Ford
Especially the XXGT and XM
Large and roomy, not too squashy
Covered in vinyl, hot and sticky

Chorus
Oh, sweet Ford of mine
Oh, sweet Ford of mine

Verse 2
As we went fast along the road
The powerful engine would roar
Because of the single or double bumper carbie
We'd go so fast we'd break the law

Chorus

Verse 3
They're good value if they're fast and have a nice interior
And are good value if they haven't clocked up much mileage
If they haven't got much rust they could last forever
The Ford Falcon I definitely our DREAM car!!!!

Final thoughts...

When helping patients with TBI to maximize their level of independence in conversations, the therapist must weigh up how much prompting and support the patient needs with how much to encourage complete independence. This is not always easy to judge. A patient's function can rapidly improve due to spontaneous recovery or it can rapidly deteriorate due to cognitive or neuroanatomical fatigue. Clinicians need to be continuously aware of these issues.

8

Assisting Children with Malignant Blood Diseases to Create and Perform their Own Songs

Trygve Aasgaard

A health perspective on song creations in paediatric cancer care

As an opening statement, it is important to state that in modern cancer care curative medical treatment has first priority. Today, carefully designed and implemented medical treatment may save the lives of the majority of children suffering from malignant blood diseases. In this process, however, the word 'cancer' and cancer-related pathology may easily overshadow any other acknowledged characteristic of the patient.

This chapter looks at songs created within the paediatric oncology environment – and sometimes beyond – from a salutogenic, ecological perspective. This does not mean that the many physical, mental and social problems related to the long periods of intensive treatment and social isolation are seen as irrelevant; they are, however, primarily understood as a backcloth for activities (and research) focusing on the health resources and health behaviour of the patient and others within the hospital community. The understanding of 'health' is here 'close to the action' – the *theoretical* position claiming that a person's health is characterized as his ability to achieve his vital goals (Nordenfelt 1987). Health is related to experiencing well-being and ability as suffering is related to experiencing disability (Nordenfelt 1987),[1] and the activities related to composing and performing potentially add health elements to the participants' lives, even at times when life itself is at stake.

In this chapter a 'song' may be understood both as a specific work of art (an object) as well as several related musical activities. Many songs are created and preserved (remembered) without being put down in writing or without ever being sung! Music is always participatory and inherently social. Song 'creations' consist of several activities that are often both enjoyable and deeply meaningful to the individual. It is one way of temporarily expanding the role repertoire of a child who seems to be 'stuck' in his or her role as a patient (one who is patiently suffering). In a broader perspective, similar activities may also normalize and 'brighten' the paediatric oncology environment (Aasgaard 2004a). This chapter demonstrates that there are different ways of assisting these patients to make and perform their own songs. The different approaches are, first of all, dependent on the child's initiatives, interests, abilities, strength and various contextual elements, such as the presence of parents in the hospital.

Limitations and challenges to music therapy activities within the paediatric oncology ward

Children with malignant blood diseases often spend several months in hospital. A common treatment programme (protocol) for Acute Lymphatic Leukaemia (ALL) lasts two years with frequent hospital admissions and periods at home where exposure to other people is very restricted. The young patients may experience both diagnostic procedures and treatment as uncomfortable, and occasionally painful. When other treatments are not effective, bone marrow transplantation offers an alternative treatment to many patients with leukaemia diseases or with related diseases (e.g. aplastic anaemia).

Occasionally chemotherapy treatment itself, like surgical interventions or radiotherapy, causes irreversible damage to vital organs. Other side effects may be uncomfortable but limited in duration, such as fatigue and pain, a sore mouth, loss of appetite, nausea, vomiting and loss of hair. Bone marrow transplantation frequently causes several complications including graft-versus-host-disease, and consequently

---

1   Nordenfelt claims that 'ability' has the advantage over 'suffering' and 'pain' of being more useful as a defining criterion for scientific and practical purposes because 'ability' to a greater extent can be intersubjectively established (1987, p.36).

the young patient often suffers more from the treatment than from the actual disease. Some of the most common stressors for the hospitalized children are related to how they are experiencing the hospital environment, where they are required to interact with strangers, and are separated from their friends or siblings during the many days of treatment and care (Melamed 1992). Several health aspects related to the young cancer patient's social relationships, self-concepts, hopes and joys are threatened, thereby restricting the young patient's possibilities for action (von Plessen 1995). Although the patients are the centre of attention and their relatives are placed at the collateral line, 'the illness' will easily dominate their lives. Professional staff working with cancer patients will also be influenced by the milieu in which they participate (Alexander 1993). Not all patients are cured, and current cancer care also reflects the limitations of modern medicine. The documented 'stories' reporting the child's musical engagement during hospitalization and artefacts thereof (such as a cassette with the child's own songs) may act as powerful testimonies about children ending their lives as something more than 'just' terminally ill cancer patients.

Technical equipment

In the mid-1990s, when I started working in hospitals with paediatric oncology wards, I used a Sony Professional cassette recorder to make cassette versions of the hospital-songs, and as I did not have access to any computerized music notation programs, all written music was produced in 'the old way'. Later notation programs like Encore, Finale and Sibelius have facilitated notation and the process of editing songs as they develop and the minidisc has taken over the task of recording the compositional process as a first step in a (potential) CD production. Today, two Norwegian hospitals have a hard disc recorder at hand for the music therapist. Hard disc recorders (properly disinfected) are also used in isolation rooms where multitrack recording sessions can take place and where the patient receives a finished CD with the song (materials) before the music therapist leaves the room. The patient also has the opportunity to create his or her own CD cover, more or less on her or his own, or as a cooperative 'family project'. However, successful songwriting projects are probably less dependent on state-of-the-art technical equipment than on music therapists being empathic, good listeners and skilled, fast working musical arrangers/accompanists, etc. But modern equipment may, indeed, increase the working capacity of the music therapist, improve the artistic products and, not the least, add elements of fun and mastery for everyone involved in the creative process.

Working methods and principles

The process of songwriting with children is inevitably flexible, and needs ⸱⸱ adapted to the needs, health situation and capacities of each individual. There are some useful guiding principles that, when considered as a way of structuring the process, provide a basic method which has guided my practice (Table 8.1).

Table 8.1 Issues and guiding principles of songwriting in child oncology

Song-related issues	Guiding principles
Promoting interest • The music therapist fostering a culture of artistic dialogues • Various song-arenas • The value of performance	• Songwriting is always voluntary and presented as a normal (cooperative) musical activity • The music therapist promotes a hospital environment with different arenas for presenting songs to others
Lyrics • What comes first? • How to get started? • Choosing a theme • Who does what?	• Individual concerns determine whether lyrics or music comes first and how to start • Indicating a specific rhythm may boost verbal processing • A well-known melody may provide a safe starting point for lyrical 'exercises' • Resist the temptation to 'take over' the making of lyrics, and never persuade the patient to choose a particular theme • Very sick children do not always prefer making songs about sickness and problems

Continued on next page

Table 8.1 (cont.)

Song-related issues	*Guiding principles*
Sound–rhythm–melody • How to get started? • Improvised playing and singing • The child's developing skills • Age appropriateness of song • Melody from rhythm – technology helps • The music therapist as composer	• 'Playing' with musical elements often initiates decision-making as to what kind of music/style the song shall have • Rhythmic features (and a specific groove or sound) may be established before the actual melody-making • When the music therapist composes a melody on his own, always think of this as a preliminary piece of art that may be rejected or altered by the patient (sooner or later)
The art of accompaniment • 'User-friendly' accompaniments • Chord symbols for accompaniments • Bass line accompaniments • Advanced accompaniments from professionals for enhancement	• When the music therapist is planning how to make an arrangement, the most important question is, 'Who is going to perform the song?' • Be careful not to 'improve' the patient's oeuvre beyond recognition; on the other hand, song arrangements and recordings that sound good are often highly appreciated by the child and the family
One song – many versions • What is useful about several versions of a song? • When the patient changes the song	• The more versions, the more fun!
Performance • Different ways of performance • The child's chosen audience • Private issues	• Songs may be too private to be performed to others; simply having made the song may be enough for the child • Playing a cassette or CD with the song to others is also a song performance

Continued on next page

Table 8.1 (cont.)

Song-related issues	Guiding principles
Songs with a long life • Why some songs become popular • The song's life outside the hospital • Sad songs • Humorous songs	• The songs with the longest lives often have a dramatic or funny story, relating to some personal experience, with simple, but well-sounding, musical elements • When the song is performed in public places, it also moves beyond the control of the young song-maker or music therapist
'Therapy' or 'project' • The 'everyday life' approach • Learning from the patients	• Making and performing songs may also be an enjoyable pastime for 'hospitalized' families • The wise therapist is always open to learn from her/his clients

Promoting an interest for songwriting

A hospital-based music therapist ought continually to strive towards developing a culture of artistic dialogues, creativity and leisure within the hospital environment. One way of being musically acquainted with the young patients also requires, when appropriate, asking their parents about *their* possible musical preferences.[2] Because patients today represent a multitude of different cultures and individual musical orientations, the music therapist often learns much from such communication which may be the very first stage of a song creative process.

Possibly the best way of inspiring the young patients to make their own songs is to provide opportunities in the ward environment where children may present their artistic works if they so wish. In the two paediatric hospital departments where I have developed music therapy services, a weekly event called the *Musical Hour* serves many purposes. This is a musical happening arranged somewhere in the open spaces

---

2   In Norway both parents are granted sick leave for as long as their child is treated for cancer. Because of this, mothers and fathers usually spend much time in the paediatric oncology ward. One father said to me that he felt it was an unwritten law that parents were held responsible for the psychosocial climate in the sick room, such as sustaining an optimistic atmosphere, and 'keeping up morale'.

(e.g. the entrance hall), and only partially pre-programmed. Here, patients, parents and hospital staff sing new or well-known songs, improvise, dramatize, get acquainted and laugh together. Often soloists, be it the medical superintendent or a ten-year-old sister of a patient, perform whatever they wish. Performing songs made in the hospital is one of many elements within this loosely structured hour of music-making with 15 or 40 participants (Aasgaard 2004a). However, the patients' rooms – even within an isolation unit – may serve as arenas for song performances. I have found that parents, nurses, doctors, teachers and other patients who demonstrate a positive interest in the songwriting business, not the least as audiences, often inspire the young artists in many ways. As a rule, the interest among the young hospitalized children for making songs seemingly appears in waves. I appreciate that this form of artistic involvement, certainly with potentially important health consequences, is not completely initiated and conducted 'from above'.

Lyrics

I present no rules as to what comes first, text or melody: a well-known text may be used as a point of departure for a new text (see Song Case 1), a text may be added to a well-known melody, the child may write a text and then participate in the musical elaboration of it (see Song Case 2) or make both a new text and a new melody to it (see Song Case 3). Many young children and teenagers want their lyrics to be based on rhymes. This is often also associated with a specific metre. If the child wants to create the lyrics within such boundaries, and then gets stuck, the music therapist may support the development of a line or verse through indicating the underlying rhythm: for example, 'tan-taran-taran-tan-tan (- . - . - - -)'. This kind of rhythmical support may be hummed or indicated on a drum or on a keyboard with hundreds of set rhythms (see Song Case 3). Young people of today often have a feeling for rap-patterns that facilitate groovy, poetic enterprises.

The easiest way of creating one's first song is to take a familiar melody or text and proceed from that starting point. In other cases it is advisable to say to the child that whichever words she or he chooses for a text, we'll get a song out of it! There have been occasions when I have suggested making a song 'from' a text – a poem or even a little story in prose style – not initially written to be sung (see Song Case 1).

I very seldom suggest a specific topic or mode of song, but tell the child (or accompanying parents) that if she or he wants to make something, I may help them if they want my assistance. I also tell them clearly what my practical contribution can be to the process, including:

- typing the text
- notating the music

- composing a melody and/or arranging the song

- recording the song

- assisting in the making of a CD cover.

An eager and result-oriented music therapist must be careful to avoid completely taking over or dominating the creative processes with which she or he is involved. At times it is tempting to suggest specific song themes relating to events or life situations which the patient is facing or already has experienced. This is a well-documented point of departure for creative-therapeutic processes where the therapist believes that making a picture/poem/song (etc.) is a good medium and activity for 'working through' one's problems and concerns. I very seldom do this or ask the child to choose between two or three thematic options, but prefer to wait for him or her to take the initiative as to 'what the song should be about' and to present the first words in the lyrics. Sometimes parents and patient collaboratively make a song text. This may result in lyrics that are mainly made by the adults; on the other hand, creative parents may teach and inspire their children to work independently as time goes on (see Song Case 1).

Sound–rhythm–melody

Similar to the process of creating 'words', music-making is a process where the music therapist continuously inspires and assists the children to present their own musical ideas. Audio-recordings of all 'sessions' are helpful to preserve any relevant musical-poetic material from one session to the next.

The grey zone between improvisation with words/musical elements and creating a song that may be reproduced is substantial. Both professional artists as well as totally untrained young composers often commence the compositional process by improvised playing or singing. If the music therapist is able to provide an unthreatening environment for sound 'doodling' and presents musical examples without predetermining the further process too much, the ignorant and apprehensive composer-to-be may begin approaching this 'serious' business with the necessary curiosity and playfulness ('playing' with sounds, rhythms and melodies). Improvisation is the common ground for developing melodies with younger children!

Young patients who observe and participate in several song-projects are likely to gradually contribute more and more to the music-making. They learn the 'tricks of the trade' as they see and hear how songs come to life. After having written nine song texts in nine months (some of them to well-known melodies), Mary is able to contribute to the melody formation for her tenth original text (Song Case 2).

Listening to recorded sessions where the music therapist explores song-related musical ideas together with the child (and sometimes members of the family) may serve as enjoyable entertainment as well as being a help to inexperienced 'composers' to develop further their ways of making music.

Composing melodies for (or together with) the more grown-up youngsters is challenging in many respects. A too 'childish' approach or result may damage the song project and even diminish the very interest for creating and/or performing the songs the music therapist is trying to nurture. Some youngsters are rather vague and unfamiliar with expressing their artistic preferences.

Case example: A 'real' teenage song

A boy of 15 who had been in the cancer ward for many months once proudly showed me his very first own song text ever. He had been helped by the hospital teacher to correct some of the many misspellings. Throughout his life, Brian had suffered many blows because of gross learning difficulties; but now he had the chance of succeeding with some 'normal' and pleasant activities. Central values in this song-project was showing the world that his song, 'Love', was made by a grown-up teenager who is writing a text about youths falling in love, and presented it in a musical rapping that other youngsters like. When we began our session of creating the music together, he could not say or do very much. His only musical recommendations were simply stating that he wanted to do 'heavy rock' and that his song must 'begin slowly'. Choosing a particular rhythm and sound on the keyboard panel initially meant more to Brian than any melodic features. (I also knew that it was most unlikely that he would ever *sing* the song himself.) His chosen style of music did not, in any way, sound 'heavy' to my ears, but Brian was blushing and stammering with pride after the first performance of 'Love' in front of the many young patients, parents and hospital staff in the audience. The words to his song were:

Love is nice girls and tough boys
loving each other.
They go to school together:
'How old are you –
can you say you love me?'
Then they move together
and that is cosy.

(Translated from the Norwegian by Trygve Aasgaard)

Many people who never manage to create a melody may easily compose some sort of rhythmic pattern. The young composer can be greatly assisted by a synthesizer, a drum machine or a keyboard with set rhythms during this stage of music-making. Even fatigued patients are often more or less capable of touching the 'drum'-keys or systematically exploring the rhythmic menu on the keyboard. When the 'right' rhythm is set, melodic rudiments or phrases may appear fairly quickly.

Case example: When a specific rhythm or sound triggers melody-making

The case example of René (p.176) presents the development of a song by a 13-year-old girl during some weeks of isolation because of potentially life-saving bone marrow transplantation. The session where the written song text became a song was, in the beginning, marked by an almost completely silent patient and an increasingly desperate music therapist proposing melodic phrases that obviously did not please the girl. Only when the music therapist started humming a rap rhythmic pattern, and the patient found the 'right' sound on the keyboard, did she begin to create some opening phrases of a melody (see Figure 8.1).

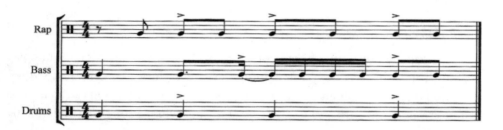

Figure 8.1 Rhythmic pattern for 'School holiday'

Within a few minutes she was whispering, singing and rapping the four verses without hesitation, using the same rap-style phrases in each verse.

When working with very sick or terminally-ill children, it may be too strenuous or time-consuming for the child to be involved in transforming a song text to a completed song. Now and then, the music therapist is, maybe partly or solely, dependent on her/his own intuition and skills when transforming a text into a song. If it is likely that the child will perform the song, the melody must be simple enough to be learnt and sung with a minimum degree of effort. The music therapist composer often balances between what may be perceived as simple, but well-sounding, melodies, and the banal or 'boring', as many children describe subjects or activities which they don't like. Once, two of my music therapy students added an incredibly swinging, but rather complicated, rock melody to a text dictated by a boy, not yet five years old (see Figure 8.2). He never managed to sing that melody properly and was not able to abstain from proceeding with the 'song' during the long pauses in the melody, but he loved listening to the students and others performing his 'nonsense' song.

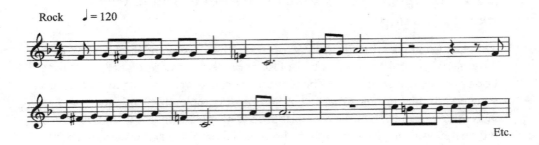

Etc.

Figure 8.2 The beginning melody of the song 'On the outside'

The art of accompaniment

Someone engaged in realizing other people's personal song projects is continuously developing the skills necessary for working with ease in various musical genres. When arranging an accompaniment for a song, the most important question is, who shall perform it? Simplicity and easiness is important when a song must be quickly learnt and performed by inexperienced musicians (see Figure 8.3). Cancer patients often lack the strength to be engaged for more than a few minutes at a time in physical activities such as singing or playing.

Although the most common way of indicating harmonic progression is by simply adding chord symbols to a melodic line, I have sometimes chosen to write a single melodic bass line (without any chords). Some children who are able to play the piano or keyboard a little may prefer this way of notation to reading chord symbols (see Figure 8.4).

As a rule, neither the child nor the family have any knowledge or interest in 'written music'. However, they may still appreciate receiving a nicely written sheet of music – some families have even framed the transcribed song and hung it on the wall like a diploma of artistic achievement.

Skilful musical accompaniments may 'turn pebbles to gold', as one mother described the 'final' recordings of her daughter's songs. Some music therapists in paediatric cancer care (for CDs with songs by children in paediatric oncology wards, see Grønnesby 2004; Köster 1997) have established contact with musicians or recording studios outside hospital to produce CD recordings where the young patient-songwriter sings accompanied by a professional musician. As an alternative to this, the music therapist may engage parents, other patients or hospital staff to take part in a performance or a recording session of a song. Depending on the patient's wishes, medical condition and degree of isolation, this may take place within the isolation room, a specially equipped music therapy room, or a room at the hospital school. Most commonly, such events cannot be planned beforehand because of the rapid changes in staff, and the many other 'more important' things going on in the ward. At any rate, it is detrimental in these situations if the music therapist attempts to make well-sounding 'manufactured' arrangements too quickly.

One song – many versions

Some young patients love to 'make' songs, but not to sing. These song makers may very much appreciate that other children or adults (such as the music therapist) will perform their productions. Other patients are temporarily not able to sing their songs; because the patient's immune system is often 'out of order', and oral mucous membranes may be sore or infected. In such cases, just trying to open the mouth may be most awkward or painful. Also the temporarily mute children appreciate hearing their songs live or recorded as soon as possible, and this necessitates making a preliminary recorded version of the song where the music therapist sings. Later, when the child has got the required strength and wish to sing, new versions may be recorded.

When the young song makers eventually leave hospital, they often have recordings of different versions of their songs. The most prolific songwriter I have met is Mary (mentioned in the clinical example on the next page and in Song Case 2). Over the course of one year in hospital she made ten songs in cooperation with the music therapist. When discharged from the hospital to go home, she received a little book with the collected original lyrics and musical arrangements. She also brought home with her a bunch of audio-tapes and a video which included at least five different versions of her most popular song 'Suspiciously cheerful' (Aasgaard 2000 and Table 8.2).

Case example: Making different versions for entertainment purposes

Once I received a small poem about 'nurses' written by a seven-year-old girl, 'Mary', who was suffering from Acute Myelogenic Leukaemia (AML). The three mentioned nurses' names corresponded with names of real nurses Mary knew;

the described activities, however, were primarily examples of Mary's newly acquired skills in rhyming!

Nurse

Inger is a star
and eats her caviar
Bodil is a star
and has a guitar
Randi is cute
and eats her soup

(Translated from the Norwegian by Trygve Aasgaard)

The bedridden girl was, at the time, neither able to sing nor to do much else. For entertainment purposes I gave the poem a melody without changing a word of it, and recorded five different versions, one 'straight' and four rather exaggerated, crazy interpretations:

1.   Straight version

2.   Punk version: with the music therapist as a not very successful punk singer accompanied by a set punk-style rhythm and related 'one-finger-on-bass' on the keyboard

3.   Cathedral version: with the music therapist chanting 'like a priest' and the keyboard in Church Organ position

4.   Jungle version: nothing but rhythmic patterns and effects from the keyboard

5.   'The dancing dolls' version: a melodic, instrumental variation based on the keyboard's 'music box' sound repertoire.

Both the girl and her parents seemed to appreciate hearing her song being 'treated' like this. Immediately after listening to the tape, Mary asked for pencil and paper, and for 15 minutes she was continuously writing, concentrating hard while remaining in absolute silence. The result was two new song texts!

I very seldom propose, change, leave out or add new words in a written or oral song text, except for 'rhythmical corrections' when one word of lesser importance is being added or removed. In texts written as prose, I sometimes repeat lines in order to make a chorus or to prolong the text at hand; a long text may also be divided to become several verses. At times, during a song performance, a child changes a melody that I have composed. The child may prefer this new version or may not be aware of her/his own alterations. A pragmatic attitude to this is simply to state that the last version is always the correct one!

Table 8.2 Five different versions of one song: 'Suspiciously cheerful'

1 (September)	A 'preliminary' recording with the music therapist singing and playing the piano. Mary was not able to sing for several months.
2 (January)	Mary singing and, here and there, spontaneously changing the melody – the music therapist accompanies on the keyboard.
3 (January)	Mary singing a version of the song where her five-year-old brother (at home) had substituted several of the original words in the lyrics with new words – all relating to farting; the music therapist accompanies on the keyboard.
4 (May)	A hospital staff choir from one of the paediatric departments performing a 'stunt' arrangement made by the music therapist who also accompanied on keyboard. When asked if she would allow the choir to sing her song, permission was swiftly granted – but Mary wants to hear the choir version (at the time she had been transferred to a different hospital).
5 (September – one year after 1)	Mary played the melody on a keyboard while the music therapist sang and played the bass-line. This session was being filmed by a major television channel.

To perform or not to perform?

Stages of creative-practical processes are neither fixed nor predetermined; sometimes several things go on at the same time. The time span between the very first idea about making a song to the completed song product may be not more than half an hour (recording included). Other songs are made within a week or two. Several things may happen to a song after its 'birth'; this is dependent on what the child-patient thinks of it, the family's interest for the song, and the music therapist's attitudes. All songs have a 'life-history' and as long as the music therapist keeps contact with the young patient, one may check out the child's interest in the songs he or she has previously made. For a variety of reasons, the child may not want to be involved with (to play/sing/talk about) a former song. The child may have strong opinions about with whom he or she wants to share his or her song. Quite often, however, the child wants to perform the song, or to play its recording, for close family members, the primary nurse, or the medical doctor. Some children also like to show their song-creating skills to other children in the oncology ward, or to classmates and friends at home. I usually ask the patients and families if they wish to have copies of the recorded song-sessions or song materials. If the patient gives the song (the CD or the written music) to his or her home school teacher (for example) to be played for, or sung to, his or her classmates, this may also be called a song performance. When families copy their hospital song audio-cassette to be given away as a Christmas gift to grandparents, etc., this is another way of performing a song to new audiences. The three Song Cases at the end of this chapter present very different stories about performing. Each song has its own 'geography' as to where it has been developed and performed (Aasgaard 2004b).

Some songs are considered as being too private to be performed to people other than the music therapist or close family members. It is important to respect the child's wishes in this respect. Only once I have said 'No, let's do this another time' to a teenager who had written a text that she wanted to share with everyone present during a 'Musical Hour'. The text was a most gloomy farewell-to-life poem addressed to her father. I believed this to be too private for the sing-song in progress, but told her that I would be happy to help her with making a melody and musical arrangement. I was later informed that the girl was not at all terminally ill! After this I never automatically interpret a song text, written in the first person singular, to be autobiographical.

Songs with a long life

The success of a song cannot be measured by counting the number of performances. But it is a fact that some songs become 'favourites' both of the song maker and various audiences. In my longitudinal studies of 19 'life histories' of songs made by children with malignant blood disorders, I have come across children who spontaneously present a new verse to a song or who show me that they now can play a song melody on an instrument many months after the completed period of treatment (see e.g. Aasgaard 2000, 2004b).[3] When other patients and relatives hear and 'learn' a song – from a live performance or from a CD – they will later use it as they like. Now the song is beyond the control of the young song maker – possibly it lives its own, indefinite life. Like any piece of art, the song may now be altered or reinterpreted to the point of being unrecognizable from the original version. Once a hospital staff rock band asked a child-composer for permission to incorporate one of her songs in

---

3   The music therapist usually has ample possibilities to meet 'old', discharged patients because of the many years of relatively frequent visits to the hospital that are needed. Many young ex-patients say 'Hello' to the music therapist and take part in some musical activity before or after scheduled medical checks in the outpatient department.

their repertoire. This is another way of expanding the audiences and the 'life length' of the song. It is not surprising that health-care workers in paediatric cancer care often find that the patients' own songs express genuine experiences, attitudes and truths that may be helpful in the education of 'the public' as well as within the professional arena.

A music therapist who is interested in the fate and therapeutic potentials of a song after it has been created will benefit from studying where and when the song was developed and used, and which people have been involved or have taken part in the song activities (audiences included). This includes obtaining information about song-related events outside scheduled music therapy sessions. The music therapist must never try to keep a song alive through 'artificial resuscitation' if the patient or family has no further interest in it. On the other hand, some songs and song-related activities seem to provide the young artists with various new and meaningful experiences for a long time. A good music therapist is one who has the skill of being a catalyst for such events to take place.

A song that is only sad and serious will seldom be used many times by the child. Such songs are often created once and only once. However, when making even the gloomiest song, this can also have elements of an achievement, making the song-writer proud and satisfied with the creative result (see Song Case 2). Songs with a funny text and a suitable, easy-to-learn melody seemingly have the greatest potentials for a long life. The combination of a dramatic text and an innocent, 'childish' melody may create or increase an ambiguous expressive message. To the song 'Suspiciously cheerful' by Mary (aged 7), the music therapist had composed a polka-like, easy-going melody. A rather violent text about a lady (a nurse or laboratory technician) who is struggling with the crying (and later fainting) patient is, indeed, a contrast to the 'happy' music (Aasgaard 2000). A common feature in several song texts is a personal, rather unpleasant experience treated in a humorous way – older children may even appreciate elements of black humour in hospital songs. Fooling doctors and nurses is almost always a popular theme, and a prominent feature of songs created by children with cancer in many situations. Griessmeier and Bossinger (1994) also describe how such songs easily become 'hits' in the paediatric oncology ward. Song Cases 1 and 3 present two different ways of using humour in a song. 'Hair poem' is probably perceived as funny because Hannah's problem of losing all her hair is being presented as solely her father's problem – a song about the harsh realities of cancer care with a sweet, little melody suitable for a song for toddlers. René's song is also full of clearly exaggerated, derogatory commentaries about her class mates…and suddenly, in the last line, we are back in the cancer ward: 'And here I am on my school holiday…'

Humour is also expressed through musical features and through particular ways of performing a song. A music therapist who is able to provide well-tailored musical solutions to the lyrics also contributes to a song product which the young song maker is proud of. On the other hand, the 'wrong' music may stop the song from being loved and used. A child will only like and use a song if both text and music is accepted as being good enough.

'Therapy' or 'project'?

In my hospital practice I present myself as the music therapist and announce my work as 'music therapy'. Only a part of my job is based on scheduled music therapy sessions in my modest office/studio. The majority of my planned individual appointments are made directly with the older child or the parents. At times I have found it practical to see families in the late afternoons or evenings and even on a Saturday or Sunday. When little else is happening, working with a song might be considered a good way of passing the time. When the song creation process has started, many interesting song-related events may take place at times when the music therapist is not present.

As a rule, I present the business of making and performing one's own songs as a musical 'project' and not as 'therapy'. I believe the meaning associated with a project is different from therapy or, indeed, a therapy *session*. Children call me 'music man', 'music therapist', 'music teacher' or 'Trygve'. Musical activities, such as making a song and performing it, are generally regarded to be within a sphere of *normality* – which I believe is not always easy to find in the high-tech environment of a university hospital. Conducting musical projects within the oncology ward is one way of demonstrating that the patients also are active, living beings. Time and time again, participating or observing parents comment that they appreciate the periods of music-making as moments when their children are temporarily leaving the patient role or hospital world. I believe it is an interesting challenge to study further how activities presented as elements of 'normal' life may have beneficial therapeutic consequences.

One good reason for applying the 'project' label on song making in the paediatric ward is simply that both the patient and the therapist may, in turn, act as 'the teacher' in the creative process. Some teenagers have quite clear ideas about the overall structure of the finished song arrangement, and they may be most willing to present and teach the music therapist some stylistic features which they think should be distinctly heard.

Case example: The patient instructing the music therapist

During a period of time during the winter I learnt how to compose songs in the 'Spice Girls' mode (which is – as a musical style – far more complex than verses and refrains presented consecutively). This case was a severely anorexic and often fatigued 14-year-old hospitalized girl who seemingly knew exactly what she wanted from me:

1. someone with whom she could discuss, test and develop her musical ideas

2. someone who could provide an accompaniment that fitted her ideas about the lyrics and music

3. someone who could record her songs.

I certainly learnt much more from this girl about composition of her chosen style of songs than she learned from me.

Parents accompanying their sick children are often knowledgeable about various musical styles and traditions and may be skilled in some musical discipline. If the music therapist always thinks cooperatively, sharing knowledge and skills easily becomes a reciprocal activity.

Case example: Hair poem

Hannah (aged 8) was suffering from aplastic anaemia; the production of healthy blood cells in the bone marrow has become most insufficient. Instead of commencing her second year at school, a bone marrow (stem cell) transplant for Hannah was planned. This was the only treatment that may help Hannah survive the rapidly progressing disease. After three-and-a-half months in one hospital, she was transferred to a new university clinic where she went through a highly aggressive chemotherapy cure before receiving a transplant of healthy bone marrow taken from her older sister (aged 15).

Four days after the transplantation Hannah became critically ill, due to an adverse reaction to cyclosporine (Zovirax), and there was an overwhelming danger of cerebral haemorrhage and that her body would reject the transplant. Hannah survived, but every day she was gradually losing her beautiful hair. One day her father picked up the shed hair…enough to fill a kidney tray. Hannah's mother is a high school lecturer and she had taken over the responsibility of being Hannah's teacher. Her father brought with him a properly disinfected guitar and, for Hannah, her descant recorder to her new home – the isolation room. Hannah's mother took the initiative to re-create a well-known Norwegian children's poem by André Bjerke, replacing the original words, but not the rhythm. Hannah was also drawn into the creative process, as she also likes to play with words. In the evening her big sister joined them and wrote down seven lines of the 'Hair poem'.

Daughter Hannah, you are funny:
you have changed your hair-style, bunny!
Father picking hair from you,
puts it in a box, quite new.
Hairless patches on your head.
Hair on floor and hair in bed.
Father's box is filled up too.

(Translated from the Norwegian by Trygve Aasgaard)

Some few days later I visited Hannah. Neither the guitar nor the recorder had been much in use lately, and that morning she had a fever over 40°C. I discovered on a table a piece of paper with 'Hair poem' written on it and immediately proposed to make a melody to it, which seemed to be a good idea. I suggested some initial phrases and Hannah sang while her father checked out chords on his guitar. When Hannah's melodic feeling and style differed from my suggestions, the phrases were therefore often altered to better match. The song was easily remembered and the accompaniment was based on only two chords. At the conclusion of this session we recorded the song with Hannah as the vocal soloist, her father on the guitar and myself playing off-beats on the treble recorder (see Figure 8.3).

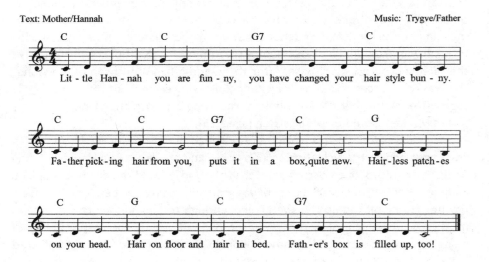

Figure 8.3 'Hair poem'

Three months later, on Christmas Eve, the Norwegian Queen visited the paediatric department. One child was designated to be her 'host' and Hannah had accepted this responsibility which also included performing a song or two. She chose to sing 'Hair poem' and another song with a text written by her mother about the bone marrow from Hannah's sister. At the big celebration she performed her song with a voice that was still brittle and weak, using a microphone and accompanied by the music therapist on a grand piano.

I met Hannah at home a couple of times after discharge and was told that the song had been performed at family parties. She now plays 'Hair poem' on the piano or recorder far more than she sings, which might suggest that developing her instrumental skills is more challenging to her than presenting a text reminding everyone about all her past problems. On the first day back at school, Hannah, together with her mother, presented slides from the isolation room and several of the hospital songs have been copied and sung in the class.

Case example: It is very boring to stay in hospital

Mary (aged 8) had been hospitalized almost a year because of Acute Myeloid Leukaemia (AML). This was a tough time for the whole family as the planned protocol of chemotherapy was not successful, and resulted in Mary being almost continuously nauseated. An aggressive, local infection resulted in the surgical removal of muscle tissue in one leg and caused much additional pain and discomfort. However, during this period she wrote several song texts and after six months she was also able to sing her songs. After receiving bone marrow taken from her little brother, her bone marrow once more functioned normally. Mary hated the immuno-suppressive medication consisting of 17, or more, big capsules to be swallowed daily. Her appetite was also poor. She was spending short periods at home, and she was allowed weekend trips to the countryside together with her family.

During one of these short stays at home, another eight-year-old girl visited Mary, and told her about all her school experiences. Mary really had nothing about school news to talk about in return, but was able at least to report that she had been creating songs. Then, as a demonstration of this skill, Mary dictated the words of her tenth song text while the friend wrote down what she said.

It is very boring to stay in hospital
It is very boring to stay in hospital
and take my medication.
And sometimes I'm throwing up,
It is not funny.
It is not funny at all.

(Translated from the Norwegian by Trygve Aasgaard)

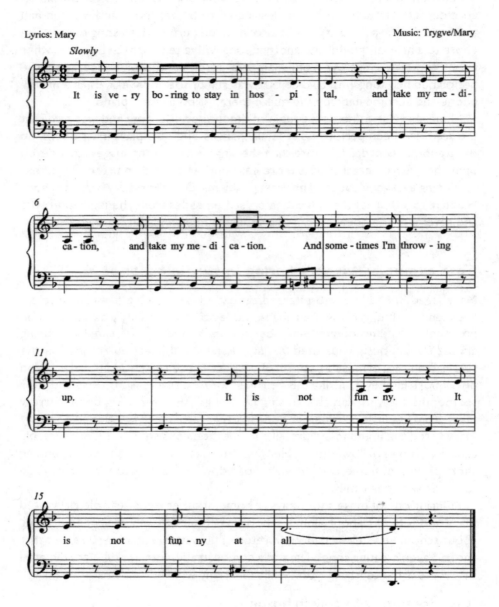

Figure 8.4 'It is very boring to stay in hospital'

The next day Mary gave me the new text (on the envelope she had written 'Song to Trygve'), and I proposed we make a melody together. She had been playing in the hospital garden for some time and was resting in bed while I am sitting at her bedside with a keyboard. She is rather passive and apprehensive at first. I suggest several opening melodic phrases and she responds to a 'falling' melodic line in the minor. Then she suggests a melody for the next line. The phrase 'and take my medication' is repeated. Within 30 minutes a melody was finished and Mary sang the entire song without accompaniment. She then changed the melody slightly, and subsequently repeated that version when we recorded the song (see Figure 8.4). Mary behaved quite 'professionally', looking relaxed and contented during the whole composition-recording session of this rather depressing song. I never heard Mary sing this song since that occasion, but some weeks later she played the melody on recorder and a mini-keyboard.

Mary's parents made the following comments about their daughter's songwriting activities:

Mother:	(about Mary's present situation at hospital) 'Just recently she called us on the mobile [telephone] and cried and was completely lost [because she had to take those medicines]. If she did not take them in the morning, she had to have a whole lot more in the evening [...] She does not vomit any longer, but she did that for a long, very long time.'
Father:	'I have a feeling that she is writing about this because she is now in fairly good shape, things have been much worse. She is actually that fit that she can be bored. She is living with numerous restrictions that were not experienced as restrictions before. She was too ill to do anything about it. This song is written in a situation where she has surplus energy to be more and to do more than sitting there, chewing tablets and becoming nauseated.'
Mother:	(about Mary and her friend)' Now their relationship is in equilibrium…actually it is Mary who is the boss.'
Father:	'Before [this event] it had been the opposite way.'
Mother:	(to the music therapist) 'I believe it has been your merit that Mary feels there is something she masters, something she is confident of and clever at. It is fantastic.'

Case example: School holiday in isolation room number nine

René (aged 13) was diagnosed as suffering from myelodysplasia when she was 12 years old. Although she had no dramatic symptoms, only bone marrow transplantation could bring a complete cure. Bone marrow from an unknown registered donor was found and her particular diagnosis necessitated a particularly tough preparation before the actual transplantation could take place. This involved an aggressive chemotherapy treatment and medicines resisting T-lymphocytes from the donor. René was admitted to hospital a week before the actual transplantation.

René's parents told the music therapist about their daughter's interest in 'making poems'. One poem had even been printed in a local newspaper. They described René as creative and resourceful. The bone marrow transplantation took place a couple of days before our first session in René's isolation room. She showed me her records and videos. Then we sang together, accompanied by me on keyboard; the refrain came from 'Give it to me, Baby' (by Offspring) and 'I'm a big, big girl'.

Three weeks after transplantation René was significantly affected by numerous side effects from the transplantation. According to her parents, she asked for a visit by the music therapist, even though she was not very fit. When I entered the room, René sat up in bed. Her eyes were closed and it seemed to be difficult for her to keep her balance when sitting. Her mouth and throat were sore, so she could only whisper or grunt. Her voice was feeble and I often had to ask her to repeat what she was trying to say. She showed me a text, in her mother's handwriting, about all the 14 other pupils in her school class at home. 'My mum has done most of it,' she said.

School holiday in isolation room number nine

I'm here in isolation room number nine,
writing a song – which is fine.
I think I'll be back in half a year,
and that day I hope everyone will cheer.

Hege, the teacher, is joking more and more,
Audun is surely the same guy as before,
Wenche is crazy and Julie's like that too,
Linn gets so angry that her face turns blue.

Kjersti is kind, and 'Tor' a nincompoop,
Trond walks about and thinks he is a 'duke'.
Geir J. and Mats both have a silly head.
They're teasing Katta till she turns red.

Vegard and Kristian are completely mad,
Thomas has a voice that is sounding sad,
Kari and Jonas are always gay,
And here I am on my school holiday.

(Translated from the Norwegian by Trygve Aasgaard)

I asked René if we should make the melody together. She said she had some ideas about how the melody ought to be. She could sing, but she was not well enough to do it just now. We decided we would wait until her voice was stronger and her throat less sore. René said, 'Do you think I could have a picture of me and you on the cover?' I answered 'Certainly.'

As agreed, I saw René in the late afternoon in order to give the text a melody. René's mother was present and, later on, her father and the primary nurse join the 'workshop'. In the beginning, René and her mother seemed rather passive, and the music therapist suggested musical phrases which René either accepted or rejected. After some time her mother exclaimed, slightly discontented: 'We have been thinking of something in rap-music style!' I started humming a rap rhythm and eventually found a convenient rhythm on the keyboard (see Figure 8.1), René started to 'rap', and within a few minutes the song had got its melody (see Figure 8.5). (René always remembered the specific numbers for the set sounds and rhythms on the keyboard.) The pitch of her hoarse voice was sometimes difficult to determine, but the rhythmical elements emerged quite distinctly. Between the verses the Primary Nurse took the initiative to sing a riff. Everyone present had a task – René: composing and rapping; Mother: commenting and singing a little; Father: technical 'engineer'; Nurse: choir-girl; Music Therapist: co-composer, musician. There was much laughter in the room during the session.

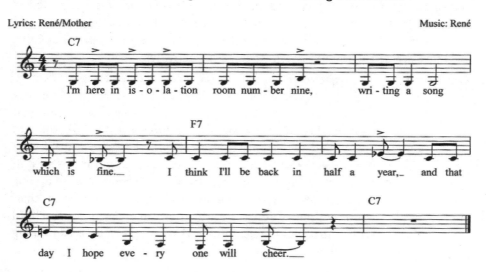

Figure 8.5 'School holiday in isolation room number nine'

It took a week before René was able to perform the song for a CD because of the very sore mucous membranes in her mouth and throat. Day by day, however, her voice gained strength. One afternoon, a microphone was placed near her mouth and René managed to rap quite well with her deep, rough, voice. Afterwards she found a picture of herself in bed while she was talking in her telephone, which at the time was considered for the cover (see Figure 8.6).

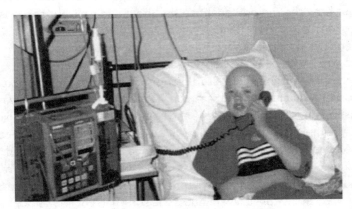

Figure 8.6 'School holiday'

The day before her transfer to a hospital 530 km away, René received two copies of her own, new CD. In her new hospital she played the CD for nurses and medical staff, and the hospital teacher played the CD for the pupils. After a couple of weeks, René called me, and asked if she could have 14 more copies of her CD (one for each pupil in her local school class). I produced the extra CDs and, on the last school day before summer vacation, the whole class was invited to René's home for a grill party. For a couple of months she had been isolated and lonely by herself at home. Now she was back and everyone got a copy of her CD.

Here are some comments on René's song activities:

Oncologist: 'It is great when children or teenagers are helped to participate in projects where they feel they really exist. For a while, as a patient, you are simply there [in the isolation room], and you feel that, broadly speaking, you do not exist. You breathe and are helped with almost everything [...] It's fantastic if, as a patient, you can be a real participant, and even more so if in addition you succeed in participating in a project like that [song creation]. We try to make life as normal as possible in 'that' room: got out of bed as soon as they can manage, doing school work and having entertainment. And this [project] is something in between.'

Father:	'This was pure fun…a way of playing with her classmates. I don't think the actual words meant that much.'
Primary nurse:	'It was exciting. It's good that this was made possible. OK, an isolation room must be tidy and clean, they are afraid of germs, etc. But we can actually think that nothing is impossible…really. […] I could see on René's face, when she found the right melody, that now it [the song] was right!'
Father:	'It was good entertainment for the family to work with this song.'
Hospital teacher:	'This CD was a good way of communication between patient and her new, temporary school, as well as between the two hospitals. René had told me that her best experience from the bone marrow treatment period was making her own CD.'
Teacher at the local school:	'René's classmates said it was astonishing and impressive that she had managed to produce something during this special situation [she had been through] and that she really had had surplus energy to give away. They also commented that the CD was so dashingly made…not looking amateurish […] and everyone was happy to receive her CD. I believe it is valuable that she was enabled to do this piece of work. I was probably not the only one who was deeply moved when listening to this song.'

Concluding remarks

My certainty as to 'what is a song' started to waver when I experienced how the young patients talked about and used their own songs: the 'content' of the song seemed occasionally to be less important than the song-related skills and activities. Studying the 'life-histories' of songs from the paediatric oncology environments widens our understanding of how children and their families *can* be artistically involved during a period of life-threatening disease, treatment and isolation. Song-creative activities are excellent expressive outlets, potentially promoting experiences of achievement and enjoyment, and are, in various ways, expanding social networks inside and outside of the hospital ward. But we still do not know if (or in what way) song activities potentially influence the trajectory of the cancer treatment.

9

Songwriting with Adult Patients in Oncology and Clinical Haematology Wards

Emma O'Brien

Introduction

Songwriting has been indicated as a highly relevant and effective therapeutic intervention with people who are undergoing treatment for cancer. Through creating a song and the resulting therapeutic relationship that develops between the patient and therapist, songwriting offers the cancer patient support during diagnosis, treatment and the palliative stages of care. Clinical reports and feedback from patients indicate songwriting as a motivating activity that can act as an outlet for held emotions and, in doing so, provide a means for the communication of thoughts and feelings that are normally difficult to express verbally. It offers an experience that is positive, aesthetic, creative and spiritual. Songwriting can offer the patient opportunities for self-expression, increased self-esteem, peace and an increased quality of life (Aasgaard 2000; Bailey 1984; Krout 2000; Lane 1988, 1992; Magill-Levreault 1993; Mandel 1991; Nolan 1992; O'Brien 1999a, 1999b, 2003; O'Callaghan 1996, 1997; Robertson-Gillam 1995; and Salmon 1993).

This chapter will offer an insight into the pathology and needs of adult cancer patients and describe how songwriting can be therapeutically applied. The method used most frequently in my practice results in writing a wholly original song. The patient is guided through the creative process creating original lyrics and original music. This method will be explained in detail and case examples will be presented to illustrate the application of the method.

The diagnosis and treatment of cancer

A diagnosis of cancer is undoubtedly a devastating experience for any individual, with consequences that impact on the individual, family and those who will become responsible as carers (Holland 1996). Treatments for cancers differ according to the nature and aetiology of the illness and the individual's presentation. All treatments have moderate to severe side effects including nausea, vomiting, loss of hair, toxicity, isolation, insomnia and pain (Coates *et al.* 1983). Most cancer patients receive several cycles of treatment and are often in hospital for extended periods of time. During these lengthy admissions they are often at risk of infection due to their lowered immune system and are consequently placed in isolation.

When diagnosed with cancer, people are faced with a crisis that affects their perception and thinking of their own mortality and meaning in their life (O'Connor, Wicker and Germino 1990). They are confronted with the physical symptoms of the disease, the prospect and consequence of ongoing treatment (Todres and Wojtiuk 1979) and the possibility of relapse (Vetesse 1976).

Post-White *et al.* (1996) explored patients' concept of hope, and strategies used to sustain it whilst facing cancer. Five recurring themes of hope were identified: finding meaning, affirming relationships, using inner resources, living in the present, and anticipating survival. Important sub-themes included faith, family, friends and future. Self-worth was described as an element in increasing patients' potential for using their inner resources as a coping strategy during treatment.

A comprehensive music therapy programme can address the multiple and complex emotional and physical needs of cancer patients (O'Brien 1999a). Music has been found to reduce patients' experience of nausea (Ezzone *et al.* 1998; Standley 1986), to reduce their anxiety (Weber, Nuessler and Wilmanns 1997), and have a positive effect on their immune system (Burns *et al.* 2001). Further, music therapy programmes can address patients' emotional and psychosocial needs (Cassileth, Vickers and Magill 2003; O'Brien 1999a, 2003; O'Callaghan 2001) by promoting well-being and relevant coping strategies during treatment.

Songwriting in cancer care

Songwriting plays a significant role in assisting self-expression and facilitating communication which leads to feelings of reduced isolation and sensory deprivation during bone marrow transplants (Hadley 1996; Lane 1992; O'Brien 2003; Robb and Ebberts 2003b). Songs created in music therapy sessions with oncology patients were helpful for newly diagnosed patients as the songs expressed commonly experienced anxieties, tensions and issues relating to cancer diagnosis and treatment (Lane 1988; O'Brien 1999b).

O'Brien (1999b) interviewed eight adult cancer patients about their experiences of songwriting and 'song sharing' in music therapy. Six of the participants were undergoing aggressive treatment for their cancers and two of the patients were in palliative care. 'Song sharing' was used as a method of intervention, which allowed the possibility for patients' own original songs to be played to others, and for patients to experience listening to other patients' songs either live or recorded. Open-ended questionnaires were used to elicit the experiences from the participants, and the themes that were identified and relevant to this chapter were:

1.   Songwriting in music therapy was a pleasurable experience.

2.   Songwriting acted as a record of a significant time in a patient's life.

3.   Songwriting was helpful in clarifying a patient's thoughts.

4.   Songwriting was a unique experience not usually expected in the hospital environment.

5.   Songwriting facilitated a positive experience of self-expression.

6.   Songwriting was a calming experience.

7.   Songwriting was an easy process, despite illness.

Undergoing a process of writing a song with another person, and creating a 'product' of a song, usually has quite an intimate quality to it, and a comfortable patient–therapist relationship was essential to address the needs of a patient through this medium of music therapy, as much as through any other.

At times songwriting methods such as word substitution, and spontaneous songs with a recognized structure (the blues), are used in my practice. However, I have found creating a wholly original song with the patient offers a depth of creative experience which can address the complexity of needs with which these patients present. It also is effective in responding to their insight orientated experiences of diagnosis and treatment. The music therapist acts as a guide offering a broad music palate and an accessible therapeutic intervention for patients (O'Brien 2003). As cancer patients can become gravely ill or, in the case of palliative patients, be terminally ill with severe side effects such as extreme pain and nausea, it is important that the method is perceived by the patients as an easy process in which to engage, despite illness (O'Brien 1999b).

The method of Guiding Original Lyrics and Music (GOLM) in songwriting

The GOLM method of songwriting has been developed in my practice over the past seven years with adult cancer patients (aged 17–85 years). It draws partly on O'Callaghan's songwriting protocol (1996) as it follows a step-by-step process and offers the patient musical examples from which to choose. The main focus of the GOLM method is on guiding the patient through the songwriting process. This method requires the therapist to be skilled in an extensive range of song styles in order to connect with the patient's individual musical expression and song genre preferences.

In the GOLM method, the patients are guided through a process which involves brainstorming ideas for the song, reframing the lyrics, delineating the style and key of the song, and in the musical setting of the lyrics. They are involved in every stage of the method.

Instruments used most regularly in my practice with this method are the guitar and voice. I have found that the guitar is a useful instrument through which to construct songs due to its versatility and capability to create a range of different musical styles. The voice is a flexible instrument, unique in its ability to convey words, melody and expression simultaneously.

When to apply the method

Creating an original song in music therapy using the GOLM method may occur as part of the natural progression of a session or may be suggested by either the therapist or the patient. The therapist may choose to instigate a songwriting session in response to issues or needs relayed by the patients, their family/carers, or the medical staff.

Within the hospital where I practise, a prevalent 'patient and therapist songwriting culture' exists. Such a culture has culminated in the production of a triple CD anthology of patient (and sometimes carer) songs (*Living Soul* 2004). Often patients have already heard other songs composed and recorded by patients and therefore the concept of songwriting within this context may not be completely novel. Despite this 'culture', songwriting is still looked upon as something someone else would do. The usual response when I suggest writing a song to a patient is, 'Oh, I could never write a song, I haven't got the talent.'

The GOLM method

The GOLM method has five stages (Table 9.1), each involving a number of considerations that the music therapist may use to guide and structure the songwriting
process.

Table 9.1 Stages in the GOLM method

GOLM stages	Guidelines and structures
1. Brainstorming	**Guiding free brainstorming and establishing rapport** **Guiding further exploration of ideas and themes**
2. Structural reframing	**Directing the free brainstorming towards a recognisable song structure** **Grouping ideas into a song structure**
3. Determining the style and key of the song	**Offering the patient different song styles** **Responding to the patient's descriptions of desired style**

4. Setting the melody and accompaniment	**Methods of guiding the melody**
	  I. Encouraging active choice
	  II. Constructing the song in sections
	  III. Deriving the organic melody
	  IV. Placing the melody into context for the patient
	  V. Integrating the patient towards creating melodies
	Notating the music in a session
	Secondary reframing of lyrics influenced by the melody
	Methods of guiding the accompaniment
	  I. Musically interpreting a patient's descriptions and/or non-verbal interactions
	  II. Spontaneously underpinning the melody
	  III. The accompaniment as a means of word painting
	  IV. Guiding the patient towards using variation within the song
	Patient's choice and ownership

5. The completed song	**Presenting and recording the finished song**

Description of the stages in the GOLM method

Brainstorming

GUIDING FREE BRAINSTORMING AND ESTABLISHING RAPPORT

In facilitating the brainstorming of ideas, the music therapist's role is to encourage patients to speak freely about any topic that interests them. It is important to let the patients know that you are not expecting them to speak in poetic or lyrical lines, and that it is not necessary for them to speak in rhyming couplets either. In the earlier stages of the session the first step is establishing rapport. This can be done using positive affirmations when the patients suggest material, and also by stimulating ideas through general conversation, which may or may not be directly related to the songwriting process. It is important to give the patients an overview of how the song will be created in a clear, non-technical manner so as to make the concept accessible.

It is the responsibility of the therapist to accurately transcribe the patients' words. Clarification through patient repetition of material may be necessary; however, the therapist should be aware that such requests may interrupt the flow of the discussion.

Gentle affirmations such as 'mmm' or 'yes' will support the patient through the initial stages of the brainstorming section and may also cue the patient to resume brainstorming ideas following a natural pause in the conversation. It is important to validate ideas offered by the patient and to remain as non-directive as possible when the patient is brainstorming freely. Towards the end of the free brainstorming section the therapist can draw upon salient comments or remarks made by the patient that can be appropriated into the developing song.

Case example: Jane's story

During the initial stages of stem cell transplantation, Jane, a 21-year-old woman with Hodgkin's lymphoma, had heard a few patients' songs during a music therapy session and was interested in writing a song. She felt a little unsure about the process, wondering about the level of difficulty required to initiate an idea. She could hardly believe that other patients had written songs, saying, 'They must have had some sort of music talent.' I reassured her at the beginning of the session by introducing the concept in approachable language.

First, we'll just have a chat about things, see if there's something you might write a song about. I'll take notes and then together we'll see what comes up. Then we can decide what might make a chorus or what we might do with the verses. Once that's sorted then we can set it to music, and basically you just tell me what you like, or sing along if something comes to you.

Jane agreed to try and the conversation began about her diagnosis. Her focus then subtly shifted to her life before that time and then quickly moved to her hopes and dreams for the future. I listened, verbally affirmed Jane's brainstorming using 'yes' and 'mmm', and I took notes. At the close of this free brainstorming section I drew Jane's attention to the three main themes that she had introduced: the experience of her diagnosis, her life before cancer and her visions for her future. Jane chose to have her future as the main focus of her song. The next stage of the session began as I commenced drawing together the ideas from the free brainstorming that directly related to Jane's hopes and dreams about her future.

GUIDING FURTHER EXPLORATION OF IDEAS/THEMES

Once the free brainstorming section has come to a natural close, exploration, reflection and confirmation of material is now the focus of the session. This is done by further exploring concepts or themes that have come up using different types of questioning. These means for the exploration of ideas are most effective when used following a direct quotation of the patient's words from the free brainstorming.

Open-ended questions are applied in the following manner to gather more general information about a theme. For example, 'You mentioned you had many dreams for your future. Could you tell me more about this?'

Direct questions are useful when trying to get more finite detail from the patient to clarify themes. For example, 'Do these hopes and dreams sustain you during this time?'

Yes, no or choice questions are useful when guiding the patient towards making a decision about his or her theme. For example, 'Would you like your song to focus on your future or your past?'

These techniques guide the patient towards deciding on a main theme for the song. While reading out loud the patient's words for clarification, I begin to group the material into common theme units. Through this guiding and grouping of the text, word strings or succinct lyric lines will be found in the direct transcription of the patient's words. Lyric lines can also evolve through further exploration and reflection of ideas.

Case example: Sandra's story

Sandra, a 45-year-old woman diagnosed with widespread pancreatic cancer being treated in palliative care, wished to write a song for her four-year-old daughter and her two older children from her previous marriage (both in their twenties). She particularly wanted the focus of the song to be directed to her youngest. She wished to include messages of everlasting love and all her dreams for her young daughter in the song. After deciding these points she was looking for a symbol of her love and care for her daughter. I began by quoting Sandra's free prose back to her and initially using an open-ended question to guide Sandra towards finding this symbol.

'Sandra, you've mentioned here that you will always be watching over your daughter. How would you like her to know this, or feel this?' Sandra responded thoughtfully, 'I'm not sure, just something she can see easily. We're not really religious, so probably not from heaven, but sort of like that. I'm not sure, but something from above.'

Sensing that Sandra wanted some sort of suggestion from me but trying to still remain open I offered her a choice question as follows. 'Would you like her to feel as if you were in the clouds, or in the stars?' Sandra instantly responded, 'I would like her to think of me as the star in the sky.' This response was noted and within the structural reframing section it became the main lyric line for the chorus of Sandra's song, 'I'll be the star in the sky'.

Structural reframing

DIRECTING THE FREE BRAINSTORMING TOWARDS A SONG STRUCTURE

At this point, as the therapist, you should become more directive in assisting the patient to focus on his/her chosen theme. Encourage the patient to think of his/her material in terms of song structure, such as chorus, verse/s, and other sections of the song. Draw together the patient's themes and words from the transcription. When reflecting what the patient has said, do so using shorter word strings, and pauses, rather than repeating it in one large body of words. This will encourage the patient to elaborate on material presented and extend his/her expression verbally. In this part of the process the patient may wish to alter his/her original words in some way, for example developing them into more poetic rhythms and metres. The role of the music therapist is important here in acting as a guide to offer solutions or variations when requested, and in assisting the patient to reframe his/her original words into lyrics. This reframing process will happen during each section of the song structure.

GROUPING IDEAS INTO A SONG STRUCTURE

Most songs have verses and a chorus. Some songs will only have verses and a refrain. Other songs will incorporate verse, chorus, bridge and refrain. How you guide the patients in structuring their song is really dependent on the material they have offered during the brainstorming section.

The *chorus* represents the major theme that has been decided upon for the song. Gather the text that expresses or supports the theme, ensuring consistent reference back to the patient for validation and confirmation. The chorus of a song often has lyric lines repeated.

The *verses* represent further explorations of the theme and may also aid in story-telling. Confirm with the patient what the role of the verses will be and then gather the information that supports this role.

The *bridge* is a connecting passage. In some cases word strings, lyrics or themes may not fit into either the verse or chorus, yet still be related to the theme of the song. Suggest to the patient at this point that these word strings or lyric lines be placed in the bridge of the song. The bridge of a song is usually set to a different melody than the chorus or verses. In the sequence of a song it can follow on from the chorus or verse, it occurs about two-thirds of the way into a song, and it often acts as a transition in the song. The bridge can incorporate modulations and as its name suggests it acts as a bridge to connect different aspects of the song. In jazz music this section of a song is often called a 'middle eight'.

The *refrain* of a song can serve a similar purpose to the chorus. It should state the main theme. It can be a truncated version of the chorus and may or may not be set to the same melody and accompaniment of the chorus.

Case example: Philip's story

Philip, a 45-year-old man with acute myeloid leukaemia undergoing a secondary salvage transplant, had found the brainstorming section very productive; to the extent that he had enough raw thematic material to create two separate songs within the session. His main themes in his session related to prayers and embracing life and Philip said that he wanted to write a song of faith, and then a more secular song. I quoted his prose and together we gathered the text that was more relevant to the sacred song surrounding his journey in prayer, and then the more secular song about looking for a brighter way in life. Philip decided that he wanted to work on the sacred song first.

Given the breadth of the information that Philip had offered, a decision as to what the focus of the chorus would be was needed. Philip decided that the chorus should be about the power of prayer. Once this theme was established he began a second level of reframing his ideas into lyrics for the chorus stating 'prayers for mercy, for faith, prayers in the morning and in the night'. I repeated his material, pausing at the end of each statement on prayers. Following the second statement Philip interjected:

> You know if you can't find an answer then one will come from above – that way people will know what I mean by all these prayers. When I lost hope I kept praying with my heart and then suddenly I had an answer, a solution.

The lyrics to the chorus were set as is illustrated below:

Prayers for mercy, pray for faith.
If you can't find an answer one comes from above.
I had no hope, I kept praying with my heart.
Suddenly a solution arrived.
Prayers in morning, prayers in the night.

When these lyrics were read to Philip in poetic metre he said he felt that it wasn't complete. He couldn't describe why, but it needed something else. I relayed back to Philip his original brainstorming word strings that related to his journey back to faith through prayer. From a group of five of his original word strings, he chose 'it helped my heart open to faith'. This line was added as the final lyric line in the chorus.

Philip wasn't sure how the verses would progress. I explained the possible general functions of verses in songs offering him the choice to either expand on his experience of prayers or to tell his story. Philip remained silent. I then revisited the original brainstorming notes and they revealed a bulk of material about his crisis of faith and how his illness had brought God back into his life. I quoted his prose and suggested using the verses to follow his journey in detail. 'Philip, you have said here, "that you had it all, but you hated yourself, and that you'd lost something in your life". Could we tell this story of loss and then how you reconnected with your prayers in the verses?' It was necessary for me to select out essential information and interpret Philip's ideas to guide him towards the structural reframing of his song. Any of the raw material that related directly to the chorus was omitted. This was done to enable the song to encapsulate the depth of Philip's expression. If I had encouraged Philip to use the verses in a similar manner to the chorus, extending on different types of prayer, the bulk of his original ideas would have not been included in the song. If a patient is not as prolific as Philip in the brainstorming phase, it may be necessary for the verses to include material which is similar to the chorus or use repetition of the lyrics in the chorus so that sufficient material is left for variation within the verses.

Patients often write songs with a listener in mind and therefore the messages within the song need to be understood by the listener. This may be a loved one, it may be other patients, or it may be the general public. If this is the case then it is the role of the music therapist to guide the patients towards making their song understood by the listener. Philip had said earlier in the session that he wanted people to learn from his experiences so he agreed to use the song as a vehicle to tell his story.

Incorporating Philip's raw material, the verses were set using a similar process of reframing as I described in the setting of the chorus. Here, Philip would offer more ideas or ask me to reframe his ideas into lyric lines. The first verse was completed.

I had it all, but I hated myself.
I'd lost the smile from my heart.
When I was a child they called me happy face,
Following my parents' steps.
So I thought I'd give it a go, and I started to pray.
Listening to God, showed me the right way.

Determining the style and key of the song

OFFERING THE PATIENT DIFFERENT STYLES

Once the patient is satisfied with the overall structure of the song, it is time to suggest setting the lyrics to music. The first step in this process is to ask the patient about his or her preferred genre of music for the song. If no specific style of music is immediately suggested by the patient, demonstrate different styles and tonalities on the guitar with verbal explanations of the examples. Initially when you are offering different options to the patients show them extremes of music styles. If you offer two very similar styles in close succession the patients may become confused and find it difficult to make a choice. When stylistic extremes are presented, the patients have a clearer understanding of the broad scope available to them and it hastens the process of finding the right sound for their song.

RESPONDING TO PATIENTS' DESCRIPTIONS OF THEIR DESIRED STYLE FOR THE SONG

It is important to describe the music in non-technical terms (avoid saying major or minor) and in so doing neutralize the 'mystique' of music composition and make it more approachable to the patient. By using more common descriptive terms such as 'sad' or 'happy', the therapist can assist the patient in identifying his or her musical preferences and interests. For musically trained and knowledgeable patients, it will be more appropriate to use musical terminology. Patients frequently indicate musical choices using descriptive terms which may describe an emotion or mood ('Can it be uplifting?') or places ('Can it sound like the sea?') or they use adjectives such as floaty, light, hard, smooth, rough, gentle and so on. Melody and accompaniment can portray these feelings and images through tonality, phrasing, melodic line, and texture. It is the music therapist's responsibility to interpret these descriptions, reflect them musically, and to confer with the patient as to whether her interpretation is an accurate representation of the patients' ideas.

Case example: Marla's story

Marla, a 26-year-old woman with acute myeloid leukaemia undergoing a bone marrow transplant, was at the stage of choosing a style for her song. Marla had chosen to write a song about turtles. Her room in the hospital was full of images of turtles, turtle ornaments and turtle toys. She said that she had always liked turtles, she found them graceful and when she heard that they were also thought to bring good luck, they had quickly become a symbol of hope, peace and positive outcomes for her during her treatment. In the lyrics of her song, Marla described why she liked turtles, but she chose not actually to say the word 'turtle'.

Verse
You seem so wise, is it because you've been here so long?
Your serene beauty brings me peace.
I just love to watch you swim; I just love to watch you swim.
I always liked you, and then I heard that you were good luck.
Your serene beauty brings me peace.
I just love to watch you swim; I just love to watch you swim.

Chorus
I can see you move as you glide through the water
It's effortless despite your size
I just love to watch you swim; I just love to watch you swim.

Marla couldn't decide on a standard style for her song. She didn't feel that a pop song suited her lyrics and she asked for something different. I began by demonstrating different styles, sound qualities and textures on the guitar with verbal explanation either proceeding or following each example. For instance I asked 'So, Marla, would you like your song to sound light?' and then I followed the question with a musical example.

Figure 9.1 illustrates the C major chord in an open position on the guitar that I played using a gentle 4/4 picking pattern, oscillating to an A minor chord in open position.

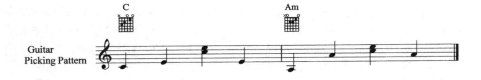

Figure 9.1 The first example of style offered by the therapist in Marla's session

When Marla's response was neutral, I changed the order of the chords and I altered my playing to a 3/4 strumming pattern and prefaced the example saying, 'Or it can start with the sad sound and then lift up.'

Figure 9.2 illustrates A minor, followed by C major, still in open position using a 3/4 strum instead of the previous 4/4 picking pattern.

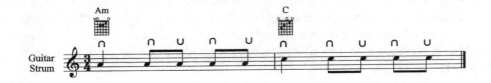

Figure 9.2 The second example of style offered by the therapist in Marla's session

Marla responded with, 'No, something different.'

I replied by offering her an extreme stylistic change. I played her a power chord, which is used in heavy rock music and shown in Figure 9.3. The power chord is derivative of a barré chord, but only the lower three notes of each chord are played. I played these with repetitive heavy down strokes on the strings. As I played this style, I spoke to Marla describing the choice I had made in response to her request, but still leaving her options open in regards to selecting a style.

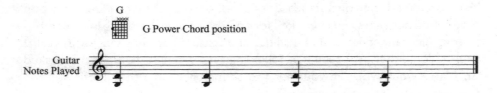

Figure 9.3 The third example of style offered by the therapist in this session

'Well would you like something more dramatic? Perhaps something that sounds harder on the guitar?...or?...[long pause]'

Marla responded to the final open question and the music example with, 'Can you make it more watery?' I musically reflected her request by playing a Bmaj⁷ chord further up the neck of the guitar using an arpeggio picking style which is commonly used in jazz music (Figure 9.4). I felt that this chord possessed watery qualities in its tonality and the arpeggio was used to accentuate this and to represent rippling waves.

Marla smiled and said, 'Yes that's it, that's the sound I want for my song.'

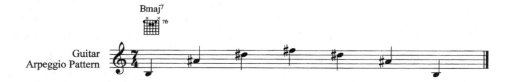

Figure 9.4 The final example of style offered in this session

On relaying this case example I realize that the reader may question why I did not automatically offer Marla this 'watery sound' in the first instance. I did this in order to provide her with the chance to arrive at the style of her song herself. I guided her through the process offering musical extremes and also framing my music examples with descriptive language. I believe that this provides patients with a strong sense of ownership of the songs and also keeps my personal music preferences and ideas secondary to theirs. Once the patient has chosen a style and key for the song, the setting of the lyrics can begin.

Setting the melody and accompaniment

Begin by explaining to the patient that once the music style is selected, further changes to the lyrics may need to be made to align with the style. When the melody is being set, it is usually derived from the lyrics, as described in the methods of guiding the melody. However, as the song progresses, the melody will begin to affect the rhythm of the lyric lines. This phase is referred to as secondary reframing.

Guiding the creation of an accompaniment may occur simultaneously with the melody; however, I have chosen to describe these two processes separately for ease of reading. Finally it is integral to the process to maintain the focus of creating the song that integrates the patient's musical expression, choices and ownership of the lyrics and music.

Methods of guiding the melody

ENCOURAGE ACTIVE CHOICE BY PATIENTS

It is important to offer the patients opportunities to contribute musically to the process through active interactions. Encourage them to be verbally directive in making selections of what they like and don't like in the music you offer to them. Assure them that a negative response to any song material that you offer will not be taken as offensive but rather brings you closer to the ultimate setting of their lyrics.

CONSTRUCTING THE SONG IN SECTIONS

Begin by setting the melody of either the chorus or the verses. This is really dependent on the pre-selected style of the song. If the song calls for a climactic chorus, it is better to begin setting the verses to allow a natural build-up into the chorus. However, in some cases, for example in many pop songs, the chorus is at the start of the song. Initially treat the song sections separately from one another to keep the process as clear as possible for the patient. Diversity between the choruses, verses, bridge and refrain are favourable for some song styles. Contrast or lack of contrast between sections will be directly effected by the lyrics and the choices made by the patient. Breaking down the songwriting process between the sections of the song reduces the possibility of the creative process as a whole appearing too daunting for the patient.

DERIVING THE ORGANIC MELODY

If the patient is happy to read aloud his or her own words (lyrics) for the song, much can be gained by listening to the natural melodic inflections in the patient's voice. If the patient is unwilling to read the text, the therapist can then read them while adopting a poetic rhythm. However, the therapist must ask for some validation from the patient to confirm that the patient likes the style the therapist is offering. Use the speech inflections in combination with the natural rhythm of the text to facilitate a melody.

PLACING THE MELODY INTO CONTEXT FOR THE PATIENT

To facilitate the creation of the melody, describe melodic lines and melodic parameters to the patient. Do this either before or after a musical example. Use hand gestures to illustrate visually the possible directions of melodic lines. This offers the patient another means of communicating his or her ideas for a melody and also encourages the patient to work towards 'conducting' (drawing out) melodies from you. Offer the patient various options for the melodic setting of the lyrics. If the patient is being non-directive begin with two melodic extremes. Melodies may be offered without accompaniment in the first instance and the accompaniment may be added later once the melodic line has been chosen; or you can underpin the melodic examples with a simultaneous accompaniment that is stylistically appropriate.

Case example: Mark's story

Mark, a 24-year-old man with acute lymphocyte leukaemia, in recovery from a bone marrow transplant, was unsure as to how his song should begin. He knew he wanted it to be a rock song, starting quietly and then building up, but he was finding it difficult to think of how the melody should sound. His song was entitled 'Pain' with the following opening lyrics:

Verse
Pain, pain it's invading me again
It hurts so much, it's driving me insane
I need a release from this pain
Oh no, not the drugs, they're in my veins
Oh the pain, the pain, the pain.

Chorus
Please release me set me free take this pain away from me. (repeated four times)

First I began to compose a melody for the verses in order to create the build-up that he wanted. He had chosen a rock style with power chords so I used them to underpin the melodic examples I was offering him. I framed each melody with a verbal description of the style and a visual representation using my right hand, before I sang and played the examples. After I asked him, 'Would you like the melody to be really still?' and simultaneously gestured a flat line, moving left to right, with my hand, I sang the first line of the verse as illustrated in Figure 9.5.

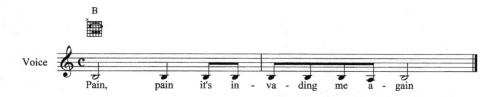

Figure 9.5 The first melodic example offered in Mark's session

Figure 9.6 shows the second example I sang to Mark, using the same lyric line, after asking him, 'Or, would you like the melody to move around a lot?', and I moved my hand vertically up and down to represent an ascending and descending melodic line.

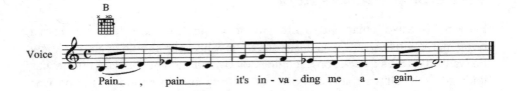

Figure 9.6 The second melodic example offered in Mark's session

After hearing both melodies Mark chose the first example shown in Figure 9.5. He qualified his choice of the static melodic line saying, 'So it [the melody] can slowly build up to the chorus', which he followed with an upward gesture, a closed fist and his extended arm. Mark continued to use hand gestures when communicating melodic choice and styles to me for the rest of the session.

INTEGRATING THE PATIENT TOWARDS CREATING MELODIES

As you move through the lyrics of the song, suggest to patients the option of repeating musical material if it is appropriate for the style of music they have chosen. For example the melody for line 1 could be repeated in line 2 or 3. Otherwise explain the possibility of creating new melodies and chord progressions for the next line of lyrics.

Encourage the patient to offer melodic examples and to complete melodic lines. This is done by singing the first line of the melody, sustaining the final note of the line and then waiting in silence to guide the patient to sing the second melodic phrase. Pausing the new melody midway through a lyric line, using sustain, then silence, can also guide the patient to complete the melodic line.

Case example: Pam's story

Despite being quite verbal during the brainstorming section, Pam, a 42-year-old woman with a rare form of lymphoma, was reluctant to offer any musical ideas for the song. When setting the lyrics to a melody I used the technique of sustaining the note and then becoming silent, either mid-phrase or at the conclusion of a melodic phrase to encourage Pam to sing a spontaneous melody. The lyrics being set in Figure 9.7 are from midway in the first verse of Pam's song and they are as follows.

They've done their job and
Now it's time
For their final farewell.

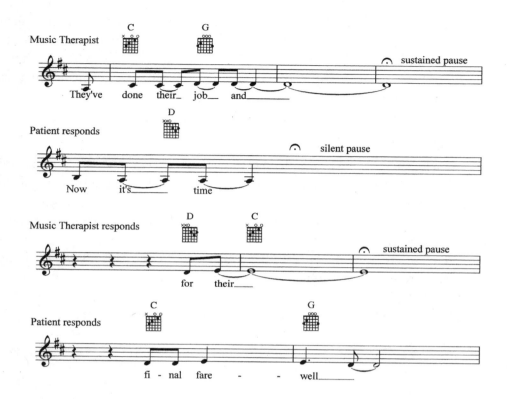

Figure 9.7 The development of an integrated melodic line using sustained notes and silence (pausing) from the therapist and melodic responses from the patient

(Pam is referring to her blood cells and how she felt about having them totally irradiated and destroyed during her chemotherapy.)

Figure 9.7 shows the development of an integrated melodic line using sustained notes and silence (pausing) from the therapist and melodic responses from the patient. It illustrates a musical dialogue between patient and therapist in the context of creating a song.

Pam continued to respond, completing many of the melodic lines in her song, progressing to singing completely new melodies, and also singing new melodies at the same time as me.

Sometimes, the therapist and patient may sing complete melodic lines simultaneously, although this tends to happen more as the session progresses and the style of the song is firmly established. For example, in popular song styles there are standard expectations of melodic resolution, and consequently the choice of genre for the song can result in pre-determined melodic structures. There is, however, a distinction between singing a new melodic line in unison, from when the patient vocally 'tracks' or follows a melody that the therapist is singing. It is often hard to distinguish between the two, so constant referring back to the patient for confirmation of melodic examples offered and chosen is important to avoid leading, as opposed to guiding, a patient's melodic expression.

Notating the music in a session

Once a melody has been selected, the therapist should sing the melody to the patient several times in order to validate his or her choice and so that the song begins to become familiar to both patient and therapist. If possible, record the session – but only for listening to later, as rewinding back to relearn new material interrupts the flow of the session. Unless the therapist is particularly skilled in notating melodies, it is useful to use a type of melodic shorthand to cue your musical memory of the song. Also be sure to notate the chords as the song progresses.

Figure 9.8 is an example of a type of melodic shorthand that I find useful in assisting me to recall melodies that have been created within the session.

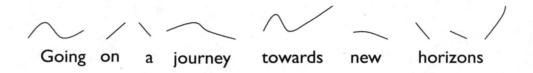

Going   on   a   journey   towards   new   horizons

Figure 9.8 An example of melodic shorthand used to notate songs during sessions

Secondary reframing of lyrics influenced by melody

Once you have set a melody to the first verse, sing the lyrics of the second verse using the same melody. If the rhythm of the music contradicts the lyrics of the second verse it may be necessary to reframe the lyrics and adapt them to fit the melodic rhythm. Returning to the original brainstorming material for word substitution or new word strings offers alternatives and maintains the integrity of the lyrics chosen. Some words may be spontaneously omitted or truncated to adjust to the melodic line. The other option is to have some variation in the melody of the second verse if the patient wants the lyrics to remain as they are. If lyrics no longer fit into the selected melodic line, but still have significance for the patient, these lyrics may be set in the bridge or refrain of the song. Discuss this possibility with the patient.

Methods of guiding the accompaniment

MUSICALLY INTERPRETING A PATIENT'S DESCRIPTIONS AND/OR PHYSICAL CUES

Patients may communicate melody by gesture (as was illustrated by my work with Mark) and/or by descriptive means. It is important to observe patients' expressive body-language as well as listening to their verbal directions. These non-verbal inter-actions can also suggest changes in accompaniment and the overall feel or mood of the song.

Case example: Pina's story

Pina, a 38-year-old leukaemia patient, re-admitted due to multiple complications after a bone marrow transplant, had song lyrics about the milestones in her life and the effect of her diagnosis and treatment on her husband, young children and extended family. We had completed the opening refrain of her song and I sang it back to her with the accompaniment on guitar (Figure 9.9). The chords are being played up the neck of the guitar with the upper four strings only in a 4/4 picking style.

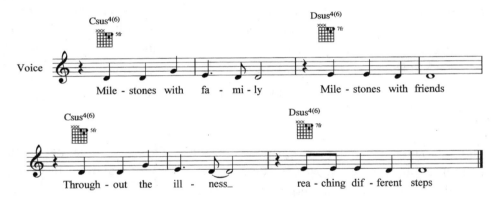

Figure 9.9 The opening melody and accompaniment to Pina's song 'Milestones'

After hearing the refrain Pina described the music as soothing, and she then requested a change in the feel of the song by gesturing in front of herself quite strongly with her fist and saying 'It [the song] needs to go here' as she held her arm and fist taut. I responded musically by moving the bass note of the chord on the guitar to the root position (on the first fret) and sang the next line of the lyrics to a melody beginning on the root note of the chord as shown in Figure 9.10.

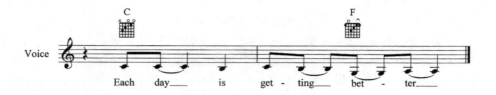

Figure 9.10 An example of interpreting a gesture and reflecting it musically during Pina's session

I musically interpreted and reflected her strong gesture as a desired move away from the 'soothing' melody and accompaniment to a more grounded chord base and strident melody. Pina affirmed the progression instantly saying, 'Yes that's it, it [that part of the song] needed more Oomph!'

SPONTANEOUSLY UNDERPINNING THE MELODY

Encourage the patient actively to choose chord progressions, where the harmonic framework will provide a relevant context for setting the lyrics to an appropriate 'musical' mood. Most patients will connect easily with the melody, and it is the therapist's responsibility to find chords that best underpin the melody chosen or spontaneously offered by the patients. Remain stylistically correct, following the genre of song style selected by the patients, unless they stipulate otherwise. Be sure to confirm all choices you make when spontaneously creating the accompaniment with the patient.

THE ACCOMPANIMENT AS A MEANS OF WORD PAINTING

At times modulations in the accompaniment may be suggested or requested by the patient using non-musical language. These chords act as a form of dramatic expression and/or word painting underpinning the specific lyrics. These choices may not be stylistically determined by the genre but provide the patient with another level of expression through the accompaniment.

Case example: Veronica's story

Veronica, 28 years of age, was at the stage of setting the melody for the first verse of her song which tells the story of her cancer relapse. She had chosen a folk ballad style in D Major and the melody for the first lyric line, 'It's something you always think is gonna happen', is shown in Figure 9.11.

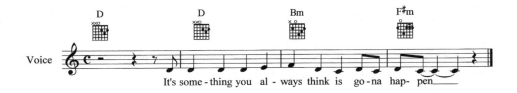

Figure 9.11 The opening melody and accompaniment to Veronica's first verse

After this melody with accompaniment had been sung back to Veronica, she requested a dramatic chord change for the next line of the verse: 'But still it's a surprise'. She wanted to set the word 'surprise' above a chord not in the standard expectation of the listener. She asked me, 'Can we really make them get a surprise in the music like I did when I found out it [the cancer] was back?'

I played her the F# Major in place of the usual tonality expected in D Major of F# minor to support her desire for detailed word painting in the song. Over this chord change I spontaneously sang a melody in a similar style to the opening melodic line as shown in Figure 9.12.

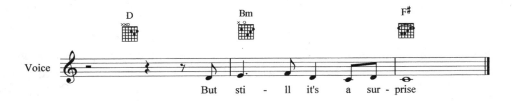

Figure 9.12 An example of word painting using the accompaniment instigated by Veronica

Veronica affirmed this use of chord word painting by clapping her hands and saying, 'Yes, now they [the listeners] will understand how I felt.'

GUIDING THE PATIENT TOWARDS USING VARIATION WITHIN THE SONG

If the patient's chosen style dictates differentiating between the verses, chorus, bridge and refrain, and this is not occurring during the natural course of setting the lyrics, it is necessary for you to guide the patients to utilize different chord progressions and melodies. As you move between the sections of the song, summarize what the patient has already completed. Describe his or her music using non-technical terms as advised earlier. When you finish setting the verses draw the patient's attention to the overall feel and sound of the song so far. For example:

> The melody in your verses is very still with a gentle guitar part underneath it; do you want the chorus to have the same feel in the melody but perhaps something different with the guitar, or would you like both the melody and the guitar to really change?

Patients may choose to keep all sections of their songs similar despite stylistic expectations. This choice needs to be validated and affirmed by the therapist even if it contradicts the chosen song genre.

Patient's choice and ownership

Patients may choose a melody or chord progression that the therapist feels is musically weak or stylistically incorrect. However, the therapist must still validate the patients' choices. Patient ownership and individual musical self-expression in the GOLM songwriting method is more important than the therapist's subjective musical opinion.

The completed song

Presenting and recording the finished song

Once the song is completed, sing it several times and encourage the patient to hum or sing along with you. If possible create an initial recording of the song for the patient to keep. Follow all appropriate ethical release forms from your organization facility to ensure that the patient is happy for his/her song to be recorded and/or heard by others. Often patients request that their songs are played live to family and friends, and they also may wish their songs to be shared with other patients and staff on the ward. Professional recordings can be made of the songs, providing you have written consent (as in the triple CD anthology we produced, *Living Soul*), to disseminate the songs to the wider public. Patients have stated that original songs created in music therapy are often more powerful and therapeutic for them than standard pop songs as they resonate with their personal experiences (O'Brien 1999b). The songs relay themes of hope, courage, love, humour and emotional responses to diagnosis, treatment and outcomes that affect people whose lives have been touched by cancer.

Adaptations of the GOLM method

Using the GOLM method with groups

I have used this method with groups of cancer patients. The stages need to be adapted in the following way to make the GOLM process accessible to the group.

BRAINSTORMING

Transcribe the brainstorming using either a whiteboard or large pieces of paper.

Do not attempt to validate every idea presented, but do try and notate them all. Try and group ideas into common themes as you transcribe their words. Keep this section of the brainstorming to a maximum of 15 minutes, taking the responsibility of drawing it to a close. When you are guiding further explorations of ideas draw the group together on the most salient theme; this will be the theme on which most of them commented in the free brainstorming.

STRUCTURAL REFRAMING

Reframe the themes into the song structure as described earlier and ask for validation of the structure from the group as a whole. Try to include at least one word string or lyric line offered by each member of the group.

DETERMINING THE STYLE AND KEY OF THE SONG

Proceed as you would with an individual patient, asking questions to the group as a whole and offering extremes of style from which to choose. Consider the average age of the group when doing this, as you would do when choosing repertoire.

SETTING THE MELODY AND ACCOMPANIMENT

With a group of adults (particularly if it is a one-off gathering) it is more likely that you will derive the organic melody from the lyrics than receive spontaneous melodic lines from individuals. Some group members will complete melodic phrases as the session progresses but they will probably request suggestions from the therapist. Maintain strong observation and listening skills to pick up on any non-verbal interactions (gesture) or descriptive language from individuals or the group. Continually place the melody and accompaniment into context for the group using non-technical terms.

The lyrics will be influenced by the melody and this secondary reframing may require you to be more directive than you would be with an individual. You are more likely to create the accompaniment spontaneously underneath their selected melodies. Guiding the group towards variation between the sections of the songs is valuable in ensuring that all the group members feel they have contributed musically to the process. You may even designate subgroups for each section of the song.

Using the GOLM method with children

I have also used this method with the children of patients. I find that at times I need to become more directive in the early stages of brainstorming to assist a child in finding a focus for his or her song (when compared to an adult), but once a style is established the melodic setting of the song is quite instantaneous, with the child either directly singing or conducting me through his or her musical ideas. The pace of the session is really determined by the age of the child and his or her concentration span. Using repetition in the song shortens the GOLM process.

The GOLM method as a dynamic process in my practice

Working as a music therapist in a public hospital places high demands on one's flexibility and diversity as a musician as the scope of patients is very broad, not only in age range but in cultures and experiences. To date I have written over 250 songs with the patients. Music styles used include: pop, jazz, funk, rock, country, grunge, techno, folk, classical, ballads, blues, R&B, soul, gospel, traditional folk, nonsense songs, rap, ambient pop, alternative, and at times an eclectic synthesis of styles.

Practising music therapy in a hospital culture also requires the ability to work efficiently in a short space of time. Over the years I have refined how I deliver this method to ensure sessions flow smoothly and that most songs are completed within an hour. I find that I am able to draw out and remember salient themes from the brainstorming as the patient is speaking, so when that section comes to a close I do not need to trawl through all my notes, which can be time consuming. I am able quickly to identify those word strings and lyric lines from the raw material which will be successful in a song and to offer alternatives to the patient, when requested, in a prompt manner. My ability to accurately interpret and reflect musically patients' non-verbal cues and descriptive non-technical terms has become more efficient. I also feel very comfortable creating spontaneous melodies and accompaniments that represent a diverse range, one after another. I have found that having a relaxed manner when approaching patients reduces their lack of confidence in their own ability to write an original song, and also helps them to trust in my experience of guiding them through the process (O'Brien 2003).

Note

All the case examples used to illustrate the method of GOLM have been sourced from my practice. In some instances names and diagnosis have been changed, but many of the patients asked for their real names and diagnosis to be revealed when talking about their songs and their songwriting experience. Permission is sought from all patients when recording their song and for their lyrics to be reproduced in music therapy sessions, for educational purposes, and in presentations.

10

The Music Therapist as Singer-songwriter

Applications with Bereaved Teenagers

Robert E. Krout

Introduction

This chapter explores the concept of the music therapist as singer-songwriter, using a didactic ten-step approach to the song composition and arrangement process. These steps are illustrated via a therapist-composed song written for use in group work with bereaved teenagers. Music therapists who write songs in and for their clinical work face many challenges. One of these is creating songs that are both clinically effective and musically interesting for their clients. While musical sophistication is not required of clients for them to benefit from songs written for them or with them by the therapist, client experiences may be enhanced and heightened when a song is musically motivating and appealing. This chapter considers one role of the music therapist as that of a singer-songwriter, in that they may create songs that weave together voice, lyrics and accompaniment to create musically interesting and clinically relevant compositions.

The image elicited by the descriptor 'singer-songwriter' may well be one of a performer such as James Taylor or Sarah McLaughlin on stage, playing and singing songs to an appreciative and involved audience. However, music therapists know that our role is not to try to be a 'performer' on stage in the clinical setting. Rather, our challenge is to involve participants in therapeutic music-based experiences to address their clinical needs and goals. As such, the title of this chapter may take some aback, as the term 'singer-songwriter' brings to mind images of MTV Unplugged. However, music therapists may accept that in songwriting, we endeavour to create songs that are musically motivating and interesting to clients, as well as being clinically sound and appropriate to their needs.

While the above concept holds true in the composition and songwriting process both for songs written by the therapist and those written by or with clients, a further challenge then becomes one of creating songs that weave voice and accompaniment together in a mutually dynamic manner to create a complete and interesting musical whole when the song is played. This is where the 'singer-songwriter' concept comes in. Rather than just providing a song accompaniment that simply musically supports the vocal line and lyrics, the 'singer-songwriter' concept brings this accompaniment to life in an active and complete arrangement. This is not to imply that all songs need complex arrangements and accompaniments. In fact, some songs will be more effective and clinically appropriate when the accompaniment is simple, especially if the client is providing the accompaniment in part or whole. For example, block chords supporting the voice may be best at times, and the therapist should not create a complex arrangement if it is clinically contraindicated or 'just because they can'.

As a preface, the theoretical and psychological orientation reflected in this chapter is what has been described in the music therapy grief literature as eclectic (Bright 2002). I see the therapist using songwriting techniques to reflect the orientation and approach they are using with any given client at that time, based on the client's needs. In addition, I have used songwriting in both individual and group music therapy, again depending on the needs of the clients at that time. The didactic approach in this chapter may be used when composing songs for group or individual music therapy.

What follows is an examination of ten considerations and techniques related to the concept of the music therapist as singer-songwriter. The song 'Be all right' will be used to illustrate each step. This particular song was written for use with grieving teenagers attending a summer grief retreat. A lead sheet for the song is shown in Figure 10.1, and I will refer to this music as each step of the process is discussed. How this song was used in the context of this group's grief work experiences will also be shared. I will begin with a brief look at songwriting in this clinical area.

Songwriting in grief work with teenagers

The use of music and music therapy in clinical interventions with bereaved children and teenagers has been described by a number of clinicians, including Dalton (1999, 2002), Dalton and Krout (2005), Hilliard (2001), Krout (2002), McFerran-Skewes and Grocke (2000), Seager and Spencer (1996), Skewes (2000), and Skewes and Grocke (2000). Specifically, songwriting has been used as a treatment modality to help children and teenagers in their grieving processes (Dalton 1999; Dalton and Krout 2005; Goldstein 1990; Hilliard 2001; Krout 2002). These interventions

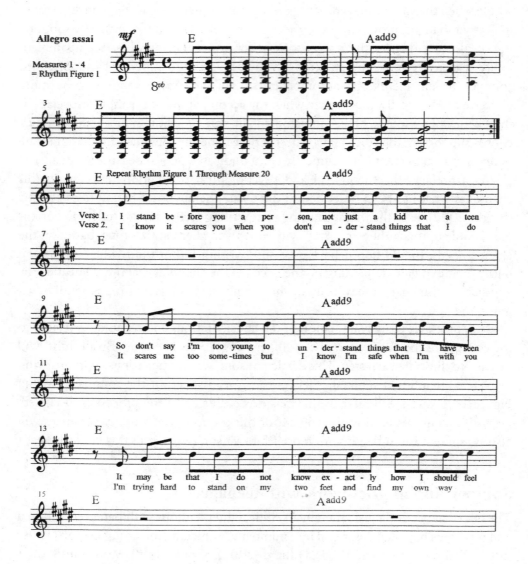

Figure 10.1 Lead sheet for the song 'Be all right'

Continued on next page

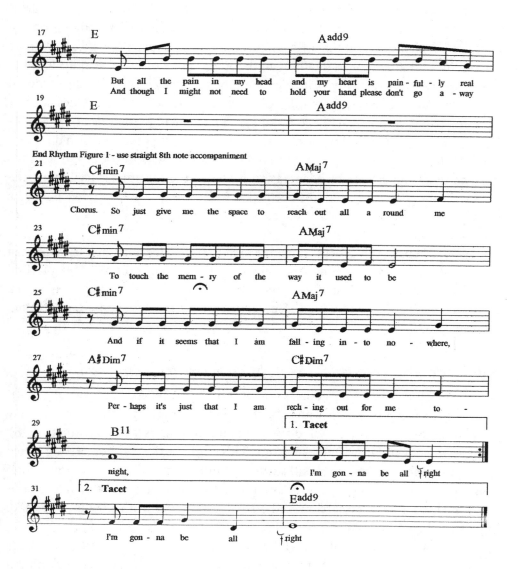

Figure 10.1 (cont.) Lead sheet for the song 'Be all right'

have included the therapist facilitating songwriting by or with the clients, as well as the therapist writing songs to be used and adapted in both individual and group music therapy grief work with children and teenagers (Bright 2002; Dalton and Krout in 2005; Krout 2002).

Using songs that the therapist has pre-composed for use in specific clinical areas such as grief interventions may be an option for the clinician, depending on the needs of the clients at that time (Krout 2004, in press[a], in press[b]). Pre-composing a song allows the therapist to incorporate the song in one or more sessions without using session time to actually write the song. The song may be used as a springboard for discussion and verbal processing, as well as for related arts activities such as drawing, painting, poetry, collage making and movement (Krout 2002).

The following is an overview of a ten-step songwriting process which describes considerations for the therapist writing the song for use in the session, although the steps and techniques may be adapted for use when the therapist is facilitating the writing of the song by or with the client(s) as well. Taking a 'step' approach may be useful in providing a system that the songwriter can follow and adapt as necessary (Blume 2004).

The ten steps in this process can be seen in overview form in Table 10.1. As can be seen, steps 1 to 3 have comments regarding the roles of both the therapist and client. Steps 4 to 10 are listed with the process steps for therapist only, as at that point the therapist is completing those steps as songwriter. I will describe each step separately.

Step 1: determine the focus of the song by examining the clinical need

Songs work best when they address one or more clinical needs or areas of significance for the client or group. Thus, the therapist must carefully consider why they are writing the song, as this will drive what kind of song is written (Brunk 1998). Some songs may be fairly simple in nature. This might be the case with a song which is used to teach or reinforce a skill such as counting or colour recognition. Other songs may be more complex, especially if they are being used to stimulate experiences such as group discussion and verbal processing with clients who have higher-level cognitive skills.

For the song 'Be all right', which I will use to illustrate this ten-step process, the needs of grieving teenagers in a bereavement setting were the factors determining the nature and focus of the song. In this case, the bereavement setting was a two-day summer programme sponsored by the Horizons Bereavement Center (HBC) of Hospice of Palm Beach County, Florida, a large hospice organization offering bereavement services to children, teenagers and adults. At the HBC, music therapy

Table 10.1 Ten steps in the songwriting process

Steps	Process steps taken by therapist in writing song	Role of client
Step 1	Determine focus of song by examining the clinical need	The clinical needs of the client(s) should drive the songwriting process. The client may be involved in this process of determining if songwriting is an experience in which they would like to be involved
Step 2	Decide who is writing song and why	Here, the therapist needs to determine if the song will be written with the client or by the therapist for use clinically with the client
Step 3	Determine which will come first, lyrics or music	At this point, and for this chapter topic, the client will not be involved in the song-writing process for this application – the pre-composing of the song for clinical use
Step 4	Rough out lyrics for content without worrying about exact word rhythm or rhyme	
Step 5	Choose style and feel for the song, using the rough lyrics as a starting point	
Step 6	Craft and design lyric rhythm and rhyme	
Step 7	Determine chords and progression and use lyrics to talk over chords	
Step 8	Add melody over chords	
Step 9	Combine 7–9 above in verse–chorus song form	
Step 10	Add additional accompaniment and stylistic features to make song unique	

components are often included in one-time grief programmes, as well as on-going grief counselling. It was called a 'retreat' for the teenagers rather than a camp, as the HBC staff had received feedback from teenager clients that calling it a camp seemed somewhat 'childish' to them.

For teenagers, music can function as a powerful catalyst for identity formation and the construction of feelings of self (Laiho 2004). As such, I wanted to write a song to help contribute to these processes within the environment of a music therapy session and the grief retreat as a whole. At the time I wrote the song, the retreat staff had an idea of how many teenagers were likely to register (about ten), their grief and loss backgrounds (included both sudden and anticipated deaths), their ages (13–16), and their genders (about even between males and females). With this information in mind, I wanted to have a song that would be appropriate to use with teenagers with a variety of backgrounds and needs. I also wanted to have a song that could be used in group work but which could also be individualized for each teenager within the group session. The overall goal of the retreat was to provide the teenagers with a safe and supportive environment in which to share about their losses and the changes in their lives since the losses. The retreat was also intended to provide interventions and experiences to help them express feelings and emotions, as well as to explore with them adaptive strategies suited to their needs.

While the retreat was not intended to substitute for on-going counselling for the teenagers, it was designed to incorporate what Teahan (2000) has termed the 'VINE' concept. These letters represent the concept of the Validation, Identification, Normalization and Expression of feelings, thoughts and emotions of bereaved children and teenagers. A goal was also to allow the teenagers to socialize, bond and have fun. The retreat was held at a beach park, Palm Beach County, Florida. In addition to a large self-contained structure with kitchen, work spaces and bathrooms, we also utilized outdoor spaces such as picnic areas, gazebos and the beach and ocean for both process-oriented experiences and recreation.

Step 2: decide who is writing the song and why

The issue of who actually writes the song is crucial and, as can be seen in this book, there are many options from which to choose. A key element is how much session time and how many sessions can be devoted to this, as a song may take several sessions to complete if working from scratch. In the case of 'Be all right', I decided to write the song before the teenager grief retreat. This song is thus an example of what Brunk (1998) terms 'strategic songwriting', which she describes as 'the process of composing a song ahead of time – for a specific goal and/or client' (p.3).

Decisions to do this were based on my plans about how to use the song in the group and on how much time was available in the session. Specifically, I planned to use this song at an early point in the retreat, in the first process group after the opening welcome. The song was thus to be the first group experience of the retreat for teenagers. I felt that starting with a receptive experience in which I played and sang the song while the teenagers first listened would be a safe experience for them. I also knew that there would be additional songwriting experiences for the teenagers at the retreat during which they could contribute to the songwriting process and have those songwriting experiences themselves.

The goal was to put some grief-related thoughts and concepts 'out there' for the teenagers to react to, and to use the song in fostering discussion regarding these concepts. In other words, this song was designed to serve as a departure point for sharing and the beginning of a group process. I did this by telling the teenagers:

> Here is a song I wrote that may relate to our weekend together and some of the things we will explore. Just listen to the song, and we can talk about it afterwards if you wish. I have copies of the lyrics if you would like them.

Step 3: determine which will come first, lyrics or music

The music therapist has choices and options as to how to begin the song creation process in terms of writing the lyrics and music. These include writing the lyrics first, composing the music first, or writing them together as the song evolves and progresses (Brunk 1998). If the therapist is writing the song with contributions from the client(s), then these options may all be available and equally valid. In fact, the clients may want to have input as to how, and in what order (lyrics, music), the song itself is created.

It is important to remember that 'Be all right' is an example of strategic songwriting (Brunk 1998) as I was writing the song ahead of time to be used in the group intervention. In the case of 'Be all right', I decided to write the lyrics first, as these would then drive the rest of my songwriting for this clinical application. In fact, the title 'Be all right' was the initial starting point for the lyrics, as it summed up the sentiment and overall message of the song. Specifically, the lyrics would influence the style, feel, chords and rhythm of the song. Again, I wanted to use the song as a springboard for verbal sharing and processing. As such, the message of the song and actual lyrics were paramount. The lyrics would form the framework of the therapeutic experience, as they would be used as the springboard for discussion and verbal processing. In addition, the music which would bring the lyrics to life as song had to reflect and work with the mood and content of the lyrics.

Step 4: rough out the lyrics for content without worrying about exact word rhythm or rhyme

Roughing out the lyrics allows the therapist to put the themes and concepts of the song into the words that the singer will communicate. Once the rough lyrics are written, the style and feel of the song may then be considered, as these will affect the lyric rhythms, chords, melody and progression. If too much time is initially spent with details such as word rhythms and rhyming patterns, the content which represents the clinical aims and goals of the song may be lost. This detail can come later and will be addressed in step 6 below.

The point of view and perspective of the singer is very important clinically, and may be the first aspect to consider. The therapist again has options, as songs may be written in the first, second or third person. In addition, the lyrics may be from a singular (e.g. 'I', 'me', 'he/she') or plural (e.g. 'we', 'they') standpoint or 'point of view'. Decisions as to these considerations should be made based on the purpose of the song clinically. With 'Be all right', the point of view is in singular first person on the part of the teenager speaking to an adult carer, who could be a surviving parent, guardian, teacher, even grief counsellor. I chose this point of view to give each teenager an opportunity to feel ownership for the lyrics if they so chose.

After this 'point of view' or 'singer's perspective' is determined, a next step is writing the lyric content, again in rough form. In a pre-composed song, this lyric content is extremely important and should represent the goals of the song as it is to be used clinically. The therapist may want to refer often to the goals they have set for the song to make sure that the lyric content is not deviating too much from that. It is easy for song lyrics to develop 'legs of their own' and wander from the intended themes.

The basic message of the 'Be all right' that I wanted to 'put out there' for the teenagers to discuss later was one related to adolescent independence combined with sharing feelings of needing support and understanding during the grief process. In addition, the message was that with this support, each teenager would find their own natural grieving process and journey to 'being all right'. I also wanted to give voice to the thoughts that the teenagers did not want to be treated as children, but to be respected as 'people'. This opinion had been shared with me by numerous teenagers in my bereavement work. I also wanted to address the theme of their wish for independence. At the same time, I wanted to reflect that it is okay to ask for help, and to seek support from adults, especially carers such as parents or guardians. Again, I wanted to write this song in the first person so that each participant could relate personally to the lyrics and have ownership of them.

Although the teenagers would not be writing the words of the song, by inviting them to listen and then discuss the lyrics and share their experiences it was hoped that the teenagers would experience some choice and control, as well as ownership of the lyrics and messages. Choice and control have been related to the concept of empowerment in music therapy with children, especially as associated with the facilitation of expression of emotions (Sheridan and McFerran 2004). Related to Teahan's VINE theme (2000), I also wanted to reinforce the message that with time and work (grief work such as that of the retreat), healing could take place for the teenagers. A number of the additional thoughts in the song have been shared with me by teenagers in my music therapy bereavement work. The following details the 'rough' lyrics, intended to provide a lyric framework without getting too particular about word rhythm or lyric rhymes:

Rough lyrics for 'Be all right'

I am my own person, not just as a 'kid' or teen
Don't talk to me like I'm a child
Don't act like I'm too young to understand that my loved one died
I don't know exactly how to feel or act, but my feelings and pain are very
   real to me
I know that you are scared sometimes when you don't understand how I
   am feeling or acting – that scares me too
I'm trying to work it out for myself – you don't need to hold my hand,
   but I do feel safe knowing you are here for me
So please, give me space to find myself
Allow me to remember my loved one and how it used to be when they
   were alive
I'm trying to figure out exactly who I am now that they have died
With time and work, it will be all right

You may want to compare these with the final lyrics below to see how they differ in final form, but not the overall message.

From these rough lyrics, I decided that the first two word groups could form verses, and that the third word group could be the chorus. These main sections of a song, the verse and chorus, are key for the singer-songwriter concept. Often the verse moves the story or plot line of a song along, while the chorus sums up the overall message of the song (Gillette 1995). The title of the song is often embedded in the chorus of a song as well, as with 'Be all right'.

Step 5: choose the style and feel for the song, using the rough lyrics as a starting point

Selecting the style and accompaniment instrument is crucial to the success of the song and the musical realization of the content of the song. The style and feel of the song should both reflect the message of the lyrics and also the music tastes and preferences of the clients. From a singer-songwriter perspective, the 'feel' of the song is of paramount importance in involving the listener in the overall mood of the song and inviting them to be 'in the moment' of that live performance of the song. In music therapy, the style and feel of a song can greatly influence how clients may respond to it (Brunk 1998).

Stylistic options are many, and include variants of folk, pop, rock, jazz, blues, contemporary, alternative, classical, show and other music. With 'Be all right', an acoustic contemporary rock feel was used. I chose this because the lyrics have a powerful message, especially as they reflect the thoughts and feelings of independence from the viewpoint of the bereaved teenagers. The contemporary rock feel was also chosen to reflect both the strength of the lyric message and the tastes of the teenagers. With the current song, the term contemporary rock refers to use of strong eighth-note (quaver) rhythms for the sung lyrics and the accompaniment, and chords that vary from the usual I, IV, V^7 and which incorporate some non-chord tones. The I (tonic), IV (subdominant) and V^7 (dominant seventh) chords are those often found in rock music, and progressions using these chords are often similar to 12 bar blues-based songs such as rock classics like 'Johnny B. Goode'. More contemporary rock songs often use more varied chords, including those not 'diatonic' to, or within, the key structure.

Another reason that I chose this stylistic feel was that I anticipated that the teenagers might have a fairly high anxiety and energy level during the first group meeting. I knew that most of the teenagers would not know each other, and that they may be nervous about the retreat and exactly what was going to happen in the groups and over the course of the weekend, etc. I wanted to have a song that could match that energy level so as to engage the group members.

The choice of accompaniment instrument is always important. Most music therapists would accompany a song with piano or guitar, although other instruments such as the autoharp and Q Chord provide alternatives. The Q Chord, which is produced by Suzuki, is a digital, portable, self-contained laptop instrument which combines features of an autoharp, piano and guitar. It uses microprocessor technology to deliver many sound and playing options. Users press chord buttons, and a rhythm section plays accompaniments in the selected musical style and tempo. The

Q Chord's 'strumplate' puts four octaves of the chord's notes at the player's finger-tips, for strumming or tapping chord notes in 100 different selectable voices.

I wrote this song to be played on acoustic guitar, which has been described as a versatile resource and base from which to write songs (Krout 2003; Rooksby 2000). The guitar is a popular instrument with teenagers (Primadei 2004; Romanowski 2003), and an acoustic guitar meant that I could play the song in almost any setting, without the need for amplification. The way a song is played also contributes to the feel, and 'Be all right' was written to be played in a singer-songwriter style that allows for a very strong guitar sound. The natural vibrations of the acoustic guitar as the primary sound source (as opposed to the amplified electric guitar) can connect the singer and the participants (Ricciarelli 2003), another aspect of the singer-song-writer approach.

Step 6: craft and design the lyric rhythm and rhyme

Step 6 is an extremely important one, as rough lyrics are transformed into lyrics with both a rhythmic pattern and a rhyme scheme. The task here is to emphasize key words based on therapeutic focus and goals, as well as to craft the rough lyrics into those which have form and rhyme schemes as desired by the therapist. The rhythm of the lyrics themselves is very important. In songwriting for therapy, the song needs of course to be singable, with sung lyric syllables accented as they would be spoken (Nordoff and Robbins 1983). However, there is also merit to accenting some lyrics 'off the beat' to add emphasis. In addition to singing the song, the therapist may want the lyrics to be spoken as well during discussion and processing with clients. This may include having the clients themselves speak some or all of the words.

In addition to word rhythm, rhyme schemes can help the listener group the lyrics together in sections, and relate lyric lines both to each other and to the song as a whole (Brunk 1998). As Blume (2004) points out, effective rhyming can help to hold the listener's attention, can help the listener remember lyrics more easily and can provide a feeling of completion and satisfaction for the listener. One standard way of rhyming words is at the end of sentences. These are known as end rhymes.

Taking this into account, I next transformed the rough lyrics for 'Be all right' from step 4 to include end rhymes. As can be seen in the final lyrics below, end rhymes happen in coupled lines – line one rhymes with line two, line three rhymes with line four, etc. The chorus has a slightly different rhyme scheme. Here, the first two lines rhyme, but the third line ends 'on its own' with the word 'nowhere'. This was done intentionally, as part of the message of the song is that, for the teenagers, it's okay to feel a bit lost sometimes. The final two lines of the chorus, which are perhaps the most important lines of the song, then rhyme.

Revised lyrics for 'Be all right'

Verse 1

I stand before you a person – not just a kid or a teen
So don't say I'm too young to understand things that I have seen
It may be that I do not know exactly how I should feel
But all the pain in my head and my heart is painfully real

Verse 2

I know it scares you when you don't understand things that I do
It scares me too sometimes but I know I'm safe when I'm with you
I'm trying hard to stand on my two feet and find my own way
And though I might not need to hold your hand, please don't go away

Chorus

So just give me the space to reach out all around me
To touch the memory of the way it used to be
And if it seems that I am falling into nowhere
Perhaps it's just that I am reaching out for me tonight
I'm gonna be all right

The word rhythms can also be seen in the lead sheet for the song (see Figure 10.1). Note the use of many repeated eighth notes (quavers). This was done to enhance the contemporary rock feel. Starting each line on the 'and' of the first beat also gives the lyrics a bit more drive.

Step 7: determine the chords and progression and use the lyrics to talk over the chords

Creating a chord progression and speaking the lyrics rhythmically over the progression helps set the feel of the song, and provides an important intermediary step to writing the actual melody. With 'Be all right', speaking the words was also designed as a possible session experience for the teenagers, as it is the lyrics which are of paramount importance. In addition, hearing and experiencing how the lyrics sound over a chord progression may give the therapist some ideas as to creating a melodic line. Of course, creating a melody first may also 'suggest' harmonies, chords and a resulting chord progression. Although I chose to start with the chords and progression before the melody, the latter may be an option for songwriters.

The therapist may also wish to have the participants speak the lyrics as well over the chord progression and accompaniment. This can be a nice way to involve participants without them having to sing. This was certainly the case with the teenagers with whom I was working, as asking a group of teenagers (who were meeting for the first time) to sing might be intimidating for them and might block group dynamics and process rather than enable them.

So, chords, a harmonic progression and an accompaniment pattern need to be selected. As can be seen in Figure 10.1, I chose E Major for the key, partly because I use guitar as the accompanying instrument for the song. Although some darker aspects of the lyrics might suggest a minor key (e.g. 'But all the pain in my head and my heart is painfully real'), I opted to use a major key, as the overall message of the song 'Be all right' is a positive one. E Major is a good strong key for guitar, with the low E and A strings giving a solid sound. This key is popular in both acoustic and electric rock music. For the verse, I selected E and A^{add9} chords. The A^{add9} was chosen for two reasons. First, it serves as the subdominant (IV) chord in the key of E. Second, the addition of the added 9th gives the chord a more open and contemporary feel. The fingering for this and all of the chords in the song can be seen in Figure 10.2.

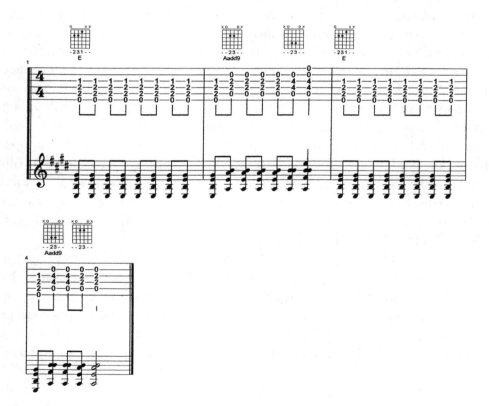

Figure 10.2 'Be all right' guitar rhythm figure

For the verse rhythm, I chose to play a variation of straight eighth notes (quavers) to provide a solid feel to the accompaniment. The variation, which can be seen in Figure 10.1, will be described in more detail in step 10. This variation is another example of the singer-songwriter approach, that of creating an accompaniment which works together with the singer to create an interesting musical whole.

The chorus, which begins on bar 21 of the song, uses more chords than the verse. For the first three lines of the chorus, I used a C# minor[7] chord and an A Major[7] chord. These are both diatonic to the key of E Major, with the Major[7] sound softening the texture a bit. The fourth line of the chorus, which is very important to the theme and message of the song, uses two diminished 7th chords to add tension. These move to a B[11] chord in the last line of the song. This chord is built off the dominant, but has a more open sound.

Step 8: add the melody over the chords

The melody brings the spoken lyric rhythms to life over the chords and progression. With the present song, the pitches chosen were designed to encourage possible singing by teenagers and to keep the melody fairly simple to emphasize the importance of the lyrics. The songwriter has many options for structuring a melody over the chords and progression. The notes available for a melody will mainly include those within the key, chord and scale structure, as well as possibly being used for colour, such as chromatic pitches which lay between these diatonic notes. If a song has key changes within it, then the available diatonic notes may change as well. Many rock songs emphasize the notes of the triads as the chords change during a progression. For instance, the rock classic 'Rock around the clock', recorded by Bill Haley and the Comets, opens with the notes of the tonic (I triad) outlined in the melody. This use of diatonic chord notes in the melody can provide stability and a stable structure for the listener, especially if they do not have extensive musical training (Radocy and Boyle 2003).

Rooksby (2000) describes the relationship between melody notes and the accompaniment harmonies as sitting inside, sitting outside of or sitting against the harmonizing notes. Melodies typically include directionality as well, and may be described in terms such as ascending, descending or arching, and may contain leaps which often resolve stepwise (Radocy and Boyle 2003). The melody can also work in tandem with the lyrics, emphasizing key words and phrases (Nordoff and Robbins 1983).

As can be seen in Figure 10.1, the melody of 'Be all right' is fairly simple, with many repeated pitches outlining the chords as above. The range of the melody is also fairly restricted, with the low note being a D, and the high note a C#. I felt that keeping the range to within an octave and not above the middle of the treble clef was important if any of the teenagers wanted to sing. The lower range also reflects the difficulties the teenagers may be experiencing in expressing themselves (e.g. 'It may be that I do not know exactly how I should feel'). A restricted range and repeated pitches are also a natural development of the spoken lyric approach described in step 7. The pitches used in the verses are higher overall than those in the chorus. This was done to give the verses and chorus a different and identifiable sound, again without stretching the overall vocal range too much.

Step 9: combine stages 7 to 9 above in verse–chorus song form

Songs and lyrics may have various combinations of verses, choruses and bridges. I opted for a simple verse–chorus–verse–chorus form to emphasize the importance of the lyrics, and to avoid getting too complicated with the song form. My goal was to involve the teenagers in the experience and song, and not to intimidate them with the complexity of it. There are many options from which to choose in putting the verses and chorus together to form a cohesive song. These are outlined in songwriting books from a number of authors, including Blume (2004), Brunk (1998), Rooksby (2000) and others. In addition to verses and the chorus, many songs have a bridge, which is a connecting passage (usually with lyrics) between the two. A bridge often serves as a release or departure from the rest of the song and can provide contrast or a different perspective (Blume 2004). In 'Be all right', I chose not to include a bridge, but rather to keep to a verse, chorus, verse, chorus form for simplicity and to help emphasize the main points and themes of the song without taking a side path.

Step 10: add additional accompaniment and stylistic features to make the song unique

This is where the singer-songwriter focus really comes in to play in making the song an arrangement which works clinically and is of musical interest to the participants. Adding unique rhythmic, harmonic and melodic elements to a song can help make it both interesting to, and motivating for, the participants and therapist. This aspect of the singer-songwriter approach is a vital element, especially when working with guitar as an accompaniment instrument. Think of songs like James Taylor's 'Fire and rain', Jim Croce's 'Time in a bottle', or Paul McCartney's 'Yesterday', and the chances are that you will think of the guitar intro first.

Additional accompaniment and stylistic elements can be rhythmic, melodic and harmonic in nature, and can include additional song features such as an intro and a coda or outro. The outro, or play-out, is an instrumental part that ends a song after the lyrics have finished. For 'Be all right', I incorporated all three of these features, which can be seen in Figure 10.1, as well as in Figure 10.3, the tablature and music notation for the guitar rhythm figure.

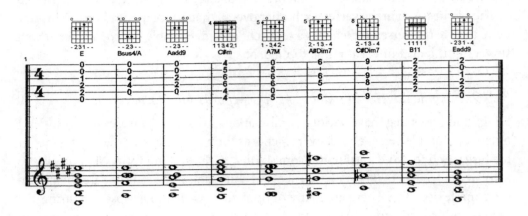

Figure 10.3 'Be all right' guitar chords

This guitar rhythm part constitutes the intro and first four bars of the song. The intro of a song is very important for therapists, as it can set the feel and mood of the song, even before the lyrics begin (Brunk 1998). The first rhythmic feature to note is the accented off-beats and groupings of eighth notes. These are intended to give the song a contemporary feeling of forward motion. A harmonic feature of the intro figure is the use of the A^{add9} chord as described in step 7 above. Note that its entrance is delayed by a half beat in each bar to coincide with the accents. Finally, a melodic element is added to the intro on the last two beats of bar 2, with the treble line moving to a high E.

This four-bar intro repeats once and then continues as the accompaniment for the verses. When the chorus begins in bar 21, a straight eighth-note (quaver) pattern is played up until bar 30, where a tacet, or break, provides a pause in the chords and accompaniment to allow the final lyric phrase 'I'm gonna be all right' to stand out. The song ends on an E^{add9} chord, designed to give the final bar an uplifted feeling.

Summary and recommendations

I used 'Be all right' with a group of teenagers at the grief retreat and it appeared to work well in facilitating a discussion of the themes. As discussed above, I introduced the song in the initial group session, offering it and the related themes within it to the teenagers for reflection and discussion. The emphasis in my presentation of the song to them was that each grief journey was uniquely theirs, but that there may be similar and common experiences and resulting feelings between each of them. The VINE-related concept that experiencing these feelings is normal was also emphasized.

After listening to and discussing the lyrics, several teenagers offered to speak lyric lines, and two asked to sing the song with me at one of the final large group meetings of the retreat. In fact, we put together an arrangement for it with some of the teens speaking or singing the lyrics, two guitars (played by me and another music therapist), and bass guitar and hand drums (played by two of the teenagers). Having the teenagers voluntarily offer to play together with me when we shared the song at the final large group meeting suggested that they had come to 'own' the song. This to me demonstrated that the song was successful in the previous stated goal of bringing the teenagers together as a group to explore issues common to their individual grief processes.

A disadvantage of the above approach might be that as the song is pre-composed by the therapist, it does not involve the clients (in this case the teenagers) in the song creation process. However, I knew that at this retreat, the teenagers would have other group songwriting opportunities. The above ten steps to creating songs from the singer-songwriter point of view may be adapted and modulated by the therapist based on the clinical needs of their clients. Additional steps could be added, again based on the clinical challenges and the therapist's own songwriting style and procedures. Please use these steps as a framework upon which to base your work and see how they function for you. The main objective is using a songwriting process to allow your creativity to be realized in songs that will help your clients with their personal and interpersonal development. As such, you may find that you use some of the above steps in a different order, for instance working on the melody before the lyrics, or developing a rhythmic pattern over which to lay the lyrics. Experiment as you wish, and don't let the above process steps inhibit your creative flow. The clinical example of the grieving teenagers at the summer retreat is one setting in which I have incorporated this songwriting model. Therapists should feel free to apply these concepts as they wish to songwriting *for* and *in* their clinical settings as well. When songwriting as or for a clinical intervention also includes the creative interplay of the singer and the accompaniment, as with the singer-songwriter concept, the therapist has in their hands and voices many options from which to choose.

11

Songwriting with Oncology and Hospice Adult Patients from a Multicultural Perspective

Cheryl Dileo and Lucanne Magill

The use of songwriting to address clinical needs of multicultural oncology and hospice patients

People experience illness and end-of-life in cultural contexts. While culture exists as a pervasive set of guidelines, both explicit and implicit, shaping the beliefs, values, feelings and behaviours of individuals (Hallenbeck 2002), it is also a dynamic process wherein people continually interact with each other, their environment and with the changing society around them. Thus, the phenomenon of culture is broad and encompasses a wide range of anthropologic, sociologic, philosophical and religious perspectives, some of which overlap and become intimately personalized according to experiences, upbringings and familial traditions. In cancer medicine and palliative care, culture seems to become even more overt, since culture plays a key role in shaping the meaning attributed to key life events, such as birth, puberty, marriage, becoming ill with a life-threatening illness, and the major life event, dying. As individuals contend with the challenge of cancer and/or terminal care, their cultural context often plays a significant role in providing a lens for perceiving and understanding the dilemma as well as a construct that provides a guide for coping, ritual and life meaning.

In oncology and palliative care, there are psychosocial, spiritual and physical ramifications of the life-threatening illness. A diagnosis of cancer can create turmoil in the life of a patient and his or her family members. Likewise, patients receiving palliative care are faced with a range of issues that can influence and have an impact upon their emotions, needs, desires, life goals and short- and long-term plans. Oncology and hospice patients and their family members are faced with losses, such as loss of self-esteem, loss of role in family or in professional duties, loss of quality time with loved ones, loss or change in physical appearance, loss or change in plans, potential loss of the hope to live a long and healthy life, loss of sense of control, and loss of financial stability and/or resources. They are also faced with transitions; for example, changes in physical energy and levels of comfort, changes in day-to-day activities and in changes in life-styles (Bailey 1984).

Patients often express the need for medical attention, emotional support, pain management, practical assistance, attention to employment and financial issues, information (Leigh and Clark 2002), and for control and spiritual support.

Patients and family members lean on many and varied coping mechanisms to get through the difficult stages of adjusting to illness and losses. Coping skills are often culturally based and are similar to the skills individuals have used throughout their lives during prior times of stress. These skills may include confrontation, finding positive aspects of the dilemma, faith, avoidance, denial or diversion. Patients and family members may be unable to cope with strong feelings due to their needs to cope with carrying on the tasks at hand. Thus, health professionals are faced with needing gently to offer empathic listening and support. Coping skills often change throughout the course of the illness and loss, especially if the patient and family members are offered non-judgemental acceptance in the supportive presence and care of health professionals.

Songwriting with multicultural oncology and hospice patients is an effective technique that provides for personalization and can offer the patient and family members opportunities to enhance communication, regain sense of control, and gain or regain a sense of fulfilment and purpose in their lives. Songwriting within their preferred cultural context can add enhanced meaning in that the songs are representative of the specific heritage, ethnicity and origin. This chapter sets out to define and describe some of the principles, practices and therapeutic methods when using songwriting with a diverse and multicultural population, in this particular case in oncology and hospice work.

Song intent

When beginning the process of songwriting with this population, patients are given the opportunity to choose the song *intent*; that is, the purpose of their song. Patients and families are invited to select the purpose and intent of their songs while also being given ample opportunity to let the song 'free-flow'; that is, to emerge naturally. Sometimes patients may choose to write a song to a loved one or to the family-at-large while expressing intimate feelings concerning the predicament. Also, patients may choose to write a song to the community or the public-at-large, to 'help others in the same situation' and as a way of giving something to others. In addition, patients may choose to dedicate a personalized song to spirituality as they know it. It is important for the therapist to let the song emerge, as the song intent may change during the course of expression, or may be multi-purposeful. There are essentially four song intents that may be developed as freely as the patient chooses:

1.   A song about one's journey: for example, song narrative, song biography.

2.   A song for a significant other, or for the surrounding family.

3.   A song for the community-at-large: for example, song dedicated to helping inspire others.

4.   A song to or for God, a Higher Power, Supreme Being or the universal, as identified by the patient.

Aims of multicultural songwriting

Multicultural songwriting in music therapy with hospitalized oncology and palliative care patients can achieve four specific aims: self-expression, relationship closure, life review and enhancement of spirituality.

Self-expression	Within a structured, yet improvisatory, framework, individuals are given the opportunity to say and express whatever they desire to say. As a result of writing a song, the patient generally experiences enhanced expression of inner thoughts and feelings that are otherwise difficult to articulate.
Relationship closure	When facing their end-of-life, individuals naturally review their lives and tend to want to come to terms with unfinished business and unresolved issues in relationships. Songwriting offers patients the opportunities to express their feelings of remorse, gratitude, hopes and appreciations. These expressions can enhance feelings of closure, often resulting in feelings of relief and resolution.

Life review   The process of life review results in the potential identification of unresolved issues as well as a review of the successes and achievements. A patient may be guided purposefully to review the stages of his/her life, as described in the song narrative section, or this may be an emergent process, as memories may begin to flow freely without therapist prompting. The therapist needs to attain a supportive demeanour in this process, since patients can sometimes become overwhelmed and/or fatigued. It is also important for the therapist to enhance a patient's sense of closure and self-esteem in this process, in order to help the patient gain a sense of satisfaction, fulfilment and sense of meaning to their life.

Enhancement of   When faced with the potential loss of life, spirituality often
spirituality   plays a significant role, as seen in the turning to faith, in the search for meaning and purpose in life, in the looking beyond the current situation to see the universal and that which exists beyond the physical, the desire to commune with nature and the significance and meaning of transcendence (Magill 2005). Songwriting affords patients opportunities to connect with, and personally express, spirituality within the context of their culture.

Multicultural issues and approaches

Besides the clinical needs of multicultural oncology or hospice patients, additional needs attributable to cultural issues often emerge. Whereas culture, defined in its broadest sense, includes many diverse factors (Dileo 2000), for the purposes of this chapter the cultural issues discussed will include only ethnicity and race. The reader is cautioned at this point to avoid over-generalizing the cultural issues presented below to specific patients, as music therapists must still approach each client as an individual who is a unique manifestation of his or her own culture.

As a general framework, world cultures may be classified as either 'individualist' or 'collectivist'. Mainstream North American and northern European cultures are often categorized as 'individualist', and Native American, Asian, Latino, African and African-American cultures are categorized as 'collectivist'.

Individualist values emphasize the role of the uniqueness of the individual who functions independently and who is responsible for him or herself as well as his or her own needs. To accomplish goals, the individual may need to exercise assertiveness and compete with others; conflict is an anticipated part of this process. The individual strives for freedom and participates as an individual democratically. He or she need not conform to others' wishes if these are in conflict with his or her own needs to self-actualize. The energy and power of youth is valued. (Dileo 2000, pp.155–6)

Alternatively, collectivist values emphasize the primacy of the group: relationships within the group and the interdependence of all within the group. Group members' first responsibilities are to the group and the group's needs.

Beyond these sweeping categorizations, specific ethnic groups may manifest specific cultural values that become quite salient when they are hospitalized with cancer or are at the end of life. These values influence the ways they cope as well as their priorities and needs. For example, Latino and Asian patients may adopt a fatalistic stance to their illness and treatment. African-Americans and Latinos, because of their inherent spiritual values, may require much spiritual support. Native American clients may cope with difficulty by withdrawal. Many of these same cultures will turn to culturally specific healing practices as alternatives to standard medical treatment. Cultural values will often determine the patient's openness to therapy; in some cultures, therapy is eschewed and highly stigmatized, and patients may turn to family, friends or religion as their primary support mechanisms. Moreover, for those cultures that are open to receiving therapy, expectations for what therapy involves may differ (e.g. being told what to do). In addition, the amount of emotional expression in response to the illness is often culturally determined; music therapists should not assume that different cultural groups will be similarly comfortable with discussing their illness-related feelings. However, the therapist may accurately assume that the patient's family structure will play a significant role in treatment and should be prepared to include these others in the treatment process.

Thus, the use of songwriting with multicultural patients may be enhanced when the patient's cultural issues are understood and acknowledged, when the music therapist is knowledgeable of song forms with which the patient may feel familiar and comfortable, and when the music therapist is flexible in addressing diverse clinical needs. To do this effectively, music therapists must: commit themselves to learning about the patient's various cultural needs and musical preferences; examine their own personal cultural values and how they may be in conflict with those of the patient; and develop authentic skills in multicultural empathy (Dileo 2000).

Cultural backgrounds are inherent aspects of the lives of oncology and hospice patients and family members. As holistic care aims to include the whole person in treatment, likewise in music therapy patients' cultural backgrounds, when considered and expanded upon in sessions, can potentially bring patients 'closer to home' and help instil enhanced feelings of peace, comfort and quality of life. Patient assessments are ongoing and fluent, due to the diverse and complex needs of oncology and hospice patients. Close attention is given to a patient's stamina and coping skills, since patients can become overwhelmed easily at times. There may be times when a patient may not have the inner strength or the desire to handle intense emotions. The therapist can help monitor the songwriting and suggest variation in the musical elements, such as rhythm and dynamics, to help the patient achieve the results he/she desires. For example, the therapist may lighten or quicken the rhythm and help the patient determine the direction and flow. Also, close attention is given to locus of control; level of pain; symptoms, such as nausea, fatigue, dyspnoea; functioning abilities; current psychosocial issues; and the needs and feelings of family members. The therapist can suggest the song intent if it is clear that certain issues could be addressed with this focus. For example, if the patient is concerned about the children who are at home, and who have been away from the parent who is the patient, the therapist may suggest writing a song for the children. Thus, patients' needs and issues are closely observed in multicultural songwriting, with the therapist attempting to become as acquainted as possible to the rituals, beliefs, values and personal perspectives of the patient's cultural background and ethnicity.

Multicultural song forms

Patient-composed songs may fulfil a variety of functions or therapeutic goals with hospitalized cancer or hospice adult patients. For example, the performance may provide a means of validating spiritual beliefs; for expressing feelings regarding the illness; for communicating needs to family, friends and staff; for self-affirmation; for life review; for finding meaning in the illness; for completing relationships; for coming to terms with death; for saying goodbye; and for leaving a song legacy.

In working with hospitalized patients with cancer or receiving hospice care, the concept of songwriting may be introduced in the first session. Except for those patients who are receiving treatments, such as bone marrow transplant, hospital stays may be relatively short in length or death may be imminent, and thus there is not an extended period of time within which a typical therapeutic rapport may evolve. At the same time, there is an inherent urgency in this type of music therapy work (Dileo and Parker 2005) because of the severity of the patient's medical condition, and the therapeutic relationship often develops quite rapidly. Because of the limited time frame within which the therapist often works and because of the patient's potential demise or discharge from the medical setting, music therapy sessions must be complete in and of themselves, with adequate resolution of issues that emerged during the session. Specifically, a song is written in its complete form usually within a single session, as there may not be another opportunity to finish it. At the same time, the therapist must be careful not to probe for deeper issues in the client that cannot be resolved within the space of a single session.

Methods used in songwriting with these clinical groups must be simple and direct. As there may not be a great deal of time to focus on the details of the music itself, the therapist may provide the musical structure, and the lyrics of the music are often afforded the primary focus. As common issues and needs are prevalent among hospitalized oncology and hospice patients, the therapist may often suggest a theme for the song lyrics, based on a discussion with the patient.

From a multicultural perspective, the music therapist should be prepared to present song forms with which the patient is familiar, and which are relevant to his or her specific culture. Song forms themselves may inherently reflect the values of the client's culture. For example, in some of the song forms from those cultures broadly termed 'collectivist' (e.g. African-American, Asian, Hispanic), one may notice several factors:

1.   Songs often involve the participation of more than one person.

2.   Songs involve improvised dialogues between or among two or more participants.

3.   Songs provide the vehicle for intense expression of emotion.

4.   Egalitarian relationships are emphasized, wherein every participant in the song has a different, yet equal, relationship to and part of the group's musical product.

5.   Call and response structures are common.

Whereas song forms from clients' own cultures may be most appropriate for use in their songwriting processes, these forms may also provide useful tools with client groups from a different culture because of their inherently 'therapeutic' structure; that is, their ability to enhance relationships, support emotional expression and facilitate direct communication.

Songwriting with multicultural client groups often involves family and friends who may be at the patient's bedside, or the patient's loved ones may often be the intended recipients of the song product. Thus, songs written may be sung by or to the therapist, the patient, the family or the staff, and according to the song's performance structure. However, the patient's physical condition is always a consideration in whether he or she is capable of singing or accompanying the song musically.

Often, the therapist will make an audio recording of the song and transcribe the lyrics for the patient and/or family. If time permits, the therapist may also transcribe the piece in musical notation.

Several song forms common to specific cultures are presented below. Due to limitations of space, this discussion is not intended to offer a comprehensive treatment of all ethnic song forms that may be relevant to music therapy songwriting practice with multicultural oncology and hospice patients. Rather, a sample of these forms is provided, and these forms may also be useful in 'traditional' music therapy practice.

The song narrative

Clients may often need to come to terms with the meaning of their lives and/or their illness through various forms of life review. The need for the patient to recount his or her own story is often pressing, and the song narrative often provides a musical structure within which this may be accomplished. Song narratives, defined for the purposes of this chapter, involve lyrics 'sung' within a very limited melodic range, on one pitch, or in rhythmic chant form. Specifically, the lyrics are performed in a type of 'spoken song' (*Sprechgesang*), a musical style that may appear more accessible to a medically frail patient. These lyrics can be supported by a chordal harmonic progression. The song structure may be strophic or through-composed, and a repetitive refrain may be employed to emphasize specific content, for example an over-arching meaning, event or person.

The composition of the lyrics for the song narrative may begin in a number of ways. The therapist may take information about the patient's life that he or she has discussed in a previous session and suggest that the client convert this into a song narrative. The therapist then may help the patient organize this information in a logical way according to a time sequence, ask the patient to freely discuss life events in a more structured way; for example, according to various chronological periods in his or her life – childhood, adolescence, adulthood. The therapist may also reflect back to the patient an overall theme that he or she has noticed in what the patient has discussed about his or her life, and this theme may be used to focus on various life events to provide a structure for the patient's story; for example, the role of spirituality in the patient's life. Alternatively, some patients may relish writing the lyrics independently, as they write their narrative history.

Once the general lyrical content is finalized, the therapist may assist the patient in organizing and condensing the words into shorter phrases or 'lines' of a stanza with a designated rhythm pattern, usually with a 4/4 metre such as that illustrated in Figure 11.1.

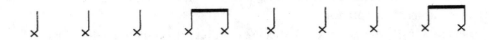

Figure 11.1 Example of rhythmic pattern of lyrics in song narratives

Stanzas may be uniform in their number of lines or not, yielding to the length of the ideas to be expressed in each. Alternatively, the song narrative may be through-composed without specific stanzas, using only the repetitive rhythm of each line as its organizing feature.

Once the lyrics have been organized rhythmically into lines, the therapist will suggest chordal accompaniment that may be consistent with the content of the lyrics.

Often simple I, IV, V progressions will be used as the basic harmonic accompaniment, and minor chords as well as diminished or augmented chords, chords with suspensions, in various inversions and with added 2nds, 7ths, 9ths, etc. may be used to reflect emotional content. If the song is organized into stanzas with the same number of lines, the chord structure may be consistent for each stanza. However, if the song is through-composed, the chords may be different for each line of the song and reflect the content of each. If a refrain is employed, a consistent harmonic accompaniment will generally be used each time it is sung.

Lyric substitution

Familiar songs can be rewritten to become personalized reflections of the patients and/or their families. This technique is cross-cultural and can be used with all ages of patients. The ease of this technique is most likely due to the fact that the song is familiar and is pre-structured, so that patients can easily and spontaneously make their own verses to identify, for example, pertinent statements about themselves, significant others, the world, their faith, their hopes, dreams and/or memories.

Any pre-composed songs can be rewritten by patients and/or family members. The therapist can use a cultural song chosen by the patient and offer to help the patient describe his/her own interpretation. Likewise, the patient may change the meaning of the song completely and use only the musical framework. The chorus can also be rewritten or can remain the same, depending on the patient's wishes as well as the patient's song intent. As with all songwriting techniques, the free-flowing improvisatory style helps the patients develop the song as it is being born.

Case example: Jim

A song, set to the tune of a mainstream North American folk song, 'Where have all the flowers gone', was created by a man in his mid-sixties, after being hospitalized for four weeks due to advanced lymphoma:

I was born in Virginia
Where all my flowers grew
Then I went to California
Where then I grew
Now I'm here with my friends and my family
It doesn't matter where I am
Just as long as we share this love
Just as long as we share this love
Just as long as we share this love.

Latino song forms

Several song forms from Latino cultures are provided as examples in this section. These forms are common in Mexico or Cuba, and have distinctive features that render them useful for therapeutic purposes.

The Mexican *ranchera* is sung in slow duple or triple metre, with simple I, IV and V^7 chordal accompaniment. In the traditional *ranchera*, the lyrics may range from sentimental to maudlin. A characteristic feature is the *grito* section where the performer may sing or speak with intense emotion (sometimes in a falsetto) (Moore 2003). The expression of intense emotion is then expected and contained within the musical structure. A familiar example of the *ranchera* is the song *Cielito Lindo*, notable for its expressive 'Ay, ay, ay, ay' chorus. This song form is useful in therapy, as it encourages and supports a description of the emotional issue in the lyrics of the verse, and then allows a direct expression of the feelings associated with the lyrics in the chorus.

In using this form in therapeutic songwriting, the therapist will usually identify a salient emotional theme needing expression as the first stage of the songwriting process. The therapist will write down and organize the patient's thoughts into fairly uniform stanzas. These are usually all written prior to the writing of the chorus. The therapist will provide a simple accompaniment as described above (or assist the client in providing his/her own accompaniment on the autoharp or guitar). After all the verses have been written and performed, the therapist will usually encourage the client to give more free expression to the feelings evoked by the verses. The therapist may suggest that these feelings be expressed through spoken word, or through singing on vowel sounds, or with words, and any combination thereof.

The Cuban *son* and *rumba* song forms are highly interactive and improvisatory. In essence, these song forms elicit spontaneous dialogues among members of a group, or between an individual and a chorus. The musical accompaniment is simple and repetitive, and provides a 'holding' function while individuals take time to organize their improvised sung statements and responses. A couplet form (two phrases) may provide the structure for the sung dialogue (Moore 2003).

In using these song forms, the therapist will often start with an initial theme that will facilitate a dialogue among the participants (e.g. patient, family, therapist). For these forms, the harmony and rhythm of the piece may be created as a starting point, and a musical couplet written or improvised. The lyrical content of this couplet may involve a provocative statement, ask a question, etc., according to the clinical theme. Once the couplet is performed, chordal accompaniment is used to 'hold the space' of the song while participants silently organize their musical responses, also in couplet form. Within this holding space, the therapist may also reflect back musically in the third person what the participant has sung, as a way of validating the individual's contribution. Couplets are usually simple melodically and rhythmically, but the initial form may be expanded or ornamented depending on the content of the response. When the song comes to a close, and there are no further improvised offerings from participants, the therapist may summarize the content of what has transpired in one or more sung couplets.

These song forms are necessarily flexible to address a number of divergent clinical issues. They may be used as a means of expressing feelings that cannot be expressed verbally, for conflict resolution, and for relationship completion (i.e. articulating love, forgiveness, thankfulness and goodbyes), among others. The emotional tone of the expressions may also range from poignant to light-hearted, even within one song.

The *Klezmer* doina

The Klezmer *doina* is typically a song of lament (and strongly influenced by religious synagogue singing) involving long sustained chords above which a voice freely improvises to express deep feelings. When sung, the *doina* may resemble a musical cry or complaint. The harmonic accompaniment is typically simple (i, iv, ii, v, i) in a minor key or in an appropriate mode (Watts 2003). It is important that the mood of the chordal accompaniment matches the mood of the improvisation. The singer may use vowel sounds or improvised words to express feelings. The vocal improvisation is usually quite ornamented, to include trills, slides, melodic suspensions, etc.

The therapist may base the vocal improvisation on a clinical issue or theme; alternatively, the client may be invited to improvise freely his or her feelings vocally. For the inexperienced client, the therapist may initially limit the number of chords used in the accompaniment and suggest a limited vocal range within which to improvise. The therapist may also demonstrate or model the song form, sing along with the client, and/or support the client vocally by singing the root of the chord he or she is playing. The therapist may use a predetermined chord structure, so the client can anticipate the change in harmony, may play the chord change while the client pauses, or may change chords to follow the client's vocalization.

African and African-American musical forms

There are several African-American song forms that may be used as structures for clinical songwriting, the most prevalent of which is the blues. The standard 12-bar blues form uses the harmonic progression illustrated in Table 11.1.

Table 11.1 Structure of the 12-bar blues form

In 4/4

Music	Lyrics
I: 3 bars	First statement of song idea
I^7: 1 bar	Usually without lyrics
IV: 2 bars	Repetition of song idea
I: 2 bars	Usually without lyrics
V^7: 1 bar	New idea, or expansion of original song idea
IV: 1 bar	Continuation of above; possible resolution of issue
I: 2 bars	Usually without lyrics

These basic chords may be altered with flattened 7ths, flat 3rds, or a variety of other harmonic and melodic ornamentations, so that an authentic 'blues' sound is achieved.

The therapist may use this song form with clients who have a need to express sadness, frustration, loneliness, pain, regret, or similar emotions, as this song form was created expressly for this purpose. Because the song form can be highly structured harmonically, and may include a great deal of repetition of lyrics, this form is quite relevant for single sessions with clients, as a complete song may be composed quite quickly.

The songwriting process begins with the identification of a theme or issue to be expressed. The therapist may help the client shape this idea into lyrics that may fit the harmonic structure. There are a number of standard blues lyric templates that may also provide structure to the lyrics (e.g. 'when I wake up in the morning…'). These lyrics may or may not be repeated in the fourth bar. In the tenth bar, while the V chord is played, a resolution to the stated issue may comprise the lyrics, or a reaction to the issue may be written, although there may be much variation to this lyric scheme. Minimally, the client may only need to compose two lines of lyrics, as the harmonic structure will already be in place. In addition, the same melody may be used for the repetition of the initial lyrics, and usually the melody will change in the tenth bar, to reflect the emotional content of the lyrics. The therapist may suggest a standard blues melody, or the client may improvise his/her own melody (Figure 11.2). The harmonic structure of the form is designed to support an infinite variety of melodies and melodic ornamentations, as well as additional words used for emphasis (e.g. 'oh, yeah'). The blues form may also be used for dialogues between

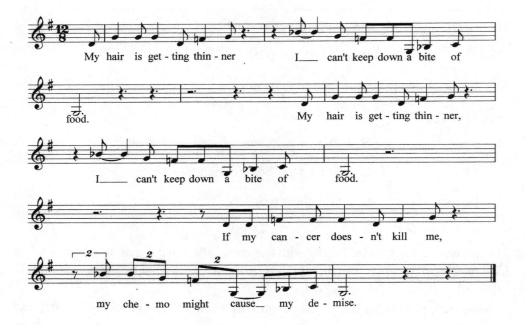

Figure 11.2 Example of a melody for a blues song

the client and therapist, wherein the therapist will provide a musical response to the idea that is presented in the 10th bar.

Call and response techniques are also common in African and African-American music. These techniques are useful musically to validate and empower the client. In using this technique, the client sings a line of a song he or she creates, and the therapist and/or family will echo back this line exactly. Alternatively, the therapist and/or family may respond with a predetermined musical line that the client has also created or may improvise new musical material. What is important in this technique is the back and forth interchange between the client and therapist/family.

Eastern Indian chants

The origins of Indian music go back far into history. Nada Brahma, which means 'the language of God', is the philosophical premise that sound is a manifestation of the divine. In Eastern Indian tradition, an Indian musician, when singing or playing, sets out to experience the infinite and to share his striving with the listener. For two thousand years, the Indian tradition of Raga Sangeet, on which the present musical system is based, has been transmitted via oral tradition, without notation, usually from father to son in lineage known as gharanas. It is one of the most sophisticated, subtle and complex musical systems in the world. Rag, tal and drone, loosely akin to melody, rhythm and a constant harmonizing background, are its basic element (Maciszewski 2000). Most rags (melodies) have specific purposes, for example to be played at certain times of the day or seasons of the year, or to promote healing, and each rag has its own principal mood or rasa. Traditionally there are nine rasas: shringara – divine or human love; hasya – humour; karuna – sadness or compassion; raudra – anger or fury; veera – heroism or majesty; bhayanaka – fear; vibhasta – disgust; adbhuta – wonder or surprise; and shanta – peace and tranquillity. Sometimes bhakti – devotion – is spoken of as the tenth rasa, but, in actuality, bhakti is a combination of the third, eighth and ninth rasas and is the very basis of rag, originating, as it did, in the singing of the Vedic chants (Maciszewski 2000).

Eastern Indian music is complex and detailed. For the purposes of multicultural work with oncology and hospice patients, the focus here is on simple chant forms. Chants play a central role in the Eastern Hindu/Vedic tradition. 'According to the sacred scriptures, The Upanishads, the cosmos was created out of the primal sound embodied in the sacred syllable "OM"' (Gass and Brehony 1999). Chants commonly uphold mantras, which are considered to be prayers, as well as 'holograms of information and energy' (Gass and Brehony 1999). There are numerous forms of chants. A simple version of Indian chant is a 16-beat pattern that repeats and ends after 32 beats. The modes of these simple chants are generally in major keys, using a I, IV, V chordal structure centred around a *tonic drone* (Table 11.2).

Table 11.2 Structure of a simple Indian chant

Music	Lyrics
I: 4 beats	Mantra
I: 4 beats	Extended or embellished mantra
I: 4 beats	Repeated mantra or continued mantra phrase
V (or IV): 4 beats	Closing mantra or continued mantra phrase

This pattern is repeated. The final four beats often conclude with an ending mantra. In this second 16-beat phase, the chords can either repeat the same first pattern, or can hold the V (or IV) for 12 beats before returning to the I. The drone continues throughout the chant. As with all chants, the 16/32 beat melodic pattern repeats for as long as a person desires.

In using this form of multicultural songwriting, the therapist can invite the patient to choose a word or group of words that are significant; that is, that can be considered to be a mantra. Since the structure of the song is created to uphold the inner being, the therapist can encourage the patient to use this format as a means of encompassing that which he/she deems meaningful. While the choice of thoughts and words is completely individual and personal, the therapist may encourage the patient to choose, for example, a special word, a thought, a prayer, a meaningful image, a personal testimony, a request, or a message for a loved one or for the universe. While chanting, the patient can be encouraged to relax and focus on the thoughts, words and images, and to allow for comfortable breathing. It is especially meaningful to have family members join in this technique, since they can offer support to the patient as well as receive support from one another. It is common for patients and families to want to incorporate the basic mantra, 'OM', into the chant, although this is always the patient's choice. The music therapist can also adapt the rhythm of the chant to the moment as a way to meet the needs of the patient. For example, the rhythm can adapt to the breathing of the patient and then can be altered, as an entrainment method, to help regulate breathing (Magill and Luzzatto 2002).

The therapist may use this song form when patients express the desire to focus their minds and thoughts. This form is also helpful with patients experiencing pain, as the repetitive pattern and the drone have lulling effects and can easily help patients relax and also potentially experience transcendence, the transporting of mind to places of beauty and tranquillity. This song form is commonly used by people of all religious and spiritual backgrounds, and is generally found to be soothing and comforting. The words selected often help patients regain a sense of control, since they are encouraged to choose words that will help them experience an enhanced sense of inner peace.

Case example: Tom

Tom, a man in his sixties with terminal cancer and in the last stage of his illness, was seen by the music therapist several weeks before his death. Tom was aware of his situation, and quite anxious about not having enough time to finish his personal business with his family. Although he had a satisfactory relationship with his wife, June, his relationship with his two grown daughters (Nancy and Sarah) was strained, and he was estranged from his son, T.J. He felt the urgent need to communicate his feelings for his family in some alternative way, as he was not able to do this by conventional verbal or written means. He saw himself as a 'no-nonsense' individual, and had worked hard during his life in the con-struction business to provide financially for his family. Because of the long hours of his work, when he returned home he was exhausted. He'd left to his wife (who was not employed) the job of caring for the children's needs and for nurturing them emotionally. He served as the disciplinarian of the house, although not severely so. He reported having rules of his home that had to be observed. Whereas his children had a warm and loving relationship with their mother, they grew to resent his emotional absence from their lives, and had not been overly attentive to him during his illness. His son held bitter feelings of resentment towards him, and made no effort to see him while he was hospital-ized.

Tom was able to express his regret to his music therapist for the decisions he had made in his life that had alienated him from his children. He wanted to feel the forgiveness of his family, and also convey to them that no matter how they perceived him as a father, he did indeed love them. The therapist suggested that Tom compose a song about his life that would convey these issues to them. Tom was not interested in having anything to do with singing, so the therapist suggested the idea of a song narrative. She stated that this type of song was similar to those of his favourite singer, Johnny Cash. As this song form was con-sistent with his culture, he agreed.

The therapist suggested that he begin with talking about his life from the time when his children were born, and then talk about various events in their lives when they were infants, children, adolescents and adults. He was asked to identify a special event for each of them that made him proud and a time when he felt especially close to each of them. He was also asked to talk about his wife and special events in their lives. As he discussed these events and feelings, the therapist took detailed notes and explored areas of emotional importance. She took particular note of certain phrases that he used repeatedly, as she felt that these would be significant in making his song narrative truly authentic. As it took a great deal of Tom's energy to recount his life story, he told the therapist that he would like her to help him organize all this material into the text for the song narrative. He was not capable of doing so. The therapist agreed, and returned several days later with a text narrative organized into strophic form. Because of his lack of physical and emotional stamina, she felt that the song should be relatively short, if he were to be able to perform it. Extracting his own words from her written notes, she organized the material into a stanza for each of his three children and one for his wife. She included a last stanza and refrain (using his own words) that helped provide closure for him and his family.

Tom decided that he would like to 'sing' the narrative in a Johnny Cash style. The therapist provided a chordal accompaniment on the guitar, and they jointly decided which chords would be appropriate for the stanzas (I– ii– V– I) and the repeating refrain (vi–I–vi I– vi I – ii V I). He instructed the therapist to use a picking pattern on the guitar which simulated a 'walking' feeling, as he walked through his life in the song. He also wanted to punctuate the refrain with percussion, hitting the cabasa with a stick. The song narrative and the chords are provided as follows:

Tom's tale
[Chords: I ii, V⁷, I for each line]

So pink, so tiny, with big blue eyes
A girl I had, my Nancy girl
Who grew to a woman, her mother's child
Yet silently in her father's heart

Sarah, you have so much of me
I 'pologize for that
From roller skates to prom queen
You've made an old man proud

My life, my son, my T.J.
You have the right to be
A man who's smart and strong
A man who's more than me

And June, my dear, my lovely bride
You did it all for me

Stood by my side and held my hand
No man could luckier be

And now as I look back at all
With tears and fears and pain
I ask you to forgive me
With love, I'll say good bye

Refrain

[vi–I–vi I– vi I – ii V I, for each line]
It takes so long for some to know all the things they have
It takes so long for some to show the feelings that were held
It may be late to right the wrongs
But try I will with my song

Tom did not want to make a live performance of this song, but asked that the therapist make a tape recording for him. The following week, he asked his wife and children to visit him in the hospital, as he knew he would soon be transferred to an inpatient hospice. His wife and daughters agreed, but his son still refused to visit him. He asked the therapist to attend this visit with his family for emotional support, and requested that she play the tape, after he provided a simple introduction to it. He told his family that this song was long overdue, and he thanked the therapist for helping him to find a way to tell them how he felt. His family listened to the tape attentively and anxiously, sometimes unable to hold back tears, especially during the verse that was dedicated to each of them. At the end of the tape, there were tear-filled smiles and laughter, as they each thanked him with a hug and told him they loved him. They joked with him about his newly discovered musical talent, and he was visibly vulnerable and tender with each of them. The moment was one of healing and transformation, one in which they found a new ending to their family history. He asked his wife to play the tape for his son, who was not present, and after having done so, his son cried, and went to see his father the following day. They had a wonderful visit that ended with an unspoken expression of love.

Case example: Ana

Ana, a 48-year-old woman, had recently been diagnosed with stage IV ovarian cancer. She had been an active career woman, a journalist and photographer, until the recent onset of difficult-to-manage pain and symptoms of discomfort. She was a wife and mother of three children, aged 10, 12 and 14. During her admission to the hospital for initial screening and treatment decisions, she was reported to be weepy and restless, pacing the floors and seeking the attention of staff. Although Ana spoke fluent English and had been living in North America for 35 years, she had cultural roots and family ties in the West Indian Islands. She was born there, and immigrated to the United States with her parents and younger sister when she was a young child. Her immediate family lived nearby; however, a large, extended family lived in her place of birth. According to staff, Ana made regular trips to the islands with her husband and children to visit her relatives. Ana was referred to the music therapist, due to her feelings of anxiety, exacerbated pain and sleep disturbance.

As the music therapist approached her in her inpatient room, Ana quickly asked her to sit down near her. She reached out her hand and asked the music therapist to stay with her for a while. She related her medical story and then began to talk about her children. She stated that she did not know what to tell them and expressed feeling very troubled about her future and the welfare of her children. She explained that her husband was very supportive; however, he was also extremely busy with his career as a business manager. She relayed her concerns for treatment schedules as well as the busy schedules of the children. She also talked at length about her desire to be with the children during their growing years. The therapist sat and listened while Ana told her story, weeping some in the process.

The therapist suggested that Ana write a song regarding her thoughts as a way to help her both express and channel some of her anxiety. Ana stated that she had 'no musical talent', but was interested in trying. The therapist asked her if she had a *song intent*. Ana said that this one would be 'just for me', since 'I know I need to take care of myself first so that I can cope with this situation and then help my family'. The therapist encouraged her to simply describe and say whatever she wanted to say, by using this time and place to help her express, ventilate and refresh herself. Ana's stamina seemed strong at this time, since she was very eager to talk and seek support. While she spoke, the therapist wrote the words down. When Ana was finished, the therapist offered to use the song style similar to a calypso. Ana smiled broadly and stated that she would be thrilled with this, as it was one of her favourite styles of music and that it always 'brings her to the homeland'. The therapist used a 4/4 rhythm with guitar strum beats alternating from a quarter note (crotchets) to two eighth notes (quavers). The therapist played a couple of simple melodies and Ana chose the one she liked. The therapist invited her to sing along, and she did. These are the lyrics to Ana's song:

Ana's home now
Built of brick now
Pigs can't knock it down
That's my home now
In Islip town

There are nine rooms there
Rather large
Four bedrooms in my home

My photographs are on the wall
Faces and places everywhere
A mosaic of my life

I like to sit in the living room
By the fire
My dog's there too

I have three children there
Treasures of mine
They miss me so much

They wish the sun would shine
I wish the sun would shine.

After Ana and the therapist completed this song, Ana smiled and appeared relaxed and noticeably calmer. The song afforded her the opportunity to channel her anxious thoughts into a melodic and rhythmic composition. The experience was cathartic for Ana, as she wept and released feelings which she had been holding on to. At the end of this session, Ana stated that she 'needed this cry' and that she felt better and more relaxed.

Three weeks later, Ana's pain had increased. She was still in the hospital, receiving chemotherapy treatments. She asked to hear songs that would help her relax while also provide her with a means for praying and focusing on 'the place of beauty that exists beyond each and every one of us'. The therapist played an Eastern Indian chant, using the 16/32 beat pattern. The therapist asked Ana to simply state whatever word or words she would like to think about, and chanted the words for her, inviting her to sing if she felt like it or to just listen and focus on the words. Ana selected the following words, and listened. The slow, even, repetitive rhythm seemed to lull her, and she closed her eyes as she listened.

Ana's chant
There is peace flowing through me [repeated three times]
Oh spirit around and within me

There is love flowing through me [repeated three times]
Oh spirit around and within me.

She also used these words: faith, beauty, sunrise and oneness.

The therapist continued to visit Ana. Together they recorded her song, at her request. Seeing that Ana seemed ready to talk with her children, the therapist asked her if she would like to now write a song for them, to express her thoughts, wishes, hopes. She was especially interested in expressing her hopes to them. The therapist offered her the popular contemporary song 'I hope you dance', suggesting that she substitute the lyrics to say whatever she wanted to say to them about her hopes. She said she loved this song and was eager to do this, especially since 'my children love to dance!' The therapist played the song without lyrics initially, and then sang the words 'I hope you...' and then paused. Ana freely filled in the pauses with her words:

Ana's song to her children
[to the tune of 'I hope you dance']

I hope you always enjoy each moment
Always know how much your mommy and daddy love you
Always be grateful for each sunrise and sunset
And laugh as often as you can.

I hope you keep faith in your hearts
Always try to do the best you can each day
Most of all, know that you are very precious
And a gift to me, your daddy and to others.

I hope you dance
I hope you dance

I hope you find the blessings all around you
And strive to reach for the good and beauty
Whether near or far, always know that I am with you
And when you get a choice to sit or dance.

I hope you dance
I hope you dance

Ana and the therapist recorded the song and Ana gave a copy to each of her children when they came to see her that weekend in the hospital. She later told the music therapist that she had a 'heart-to-heart' talk with them that day as she gave them each a copy of the recording. She felt relieved to have shared with them that she was quite ill and would not be home for a while. As she had planned, she played the recording for them while they sat next to her on her bed. They shared moments of tears, laughter and love while the husband held her hand. The song facilitated and provided for moments of healing for Ana, her children and her husband, as they each were able to express their love for each other.

Conclusion

The issues of oncology and hospice patients are complex and numerous, and the issue of culture imposes another layer for clinical consideration. The culturally sensitive music therapist is challenged musically, intellectually and personally. As songwriting may provide a meaningful intervention in helping patients express and ultimately come to terms with what they are facing, music therapists must possess extraordinary sensitivity, compassion and flexibility. In addition, they need to be prepared for this work with knowledge of and skill in ethnic song forms, knowledge of potential cultural characteristics, and a keen sense of their own cultural attitudes and biases. When skilled in this way, the therapist may facilitate and witness unforgettably poignant and transformative experiences that impact deeply upon the critical and final moments of patients' lives.

12

Songwriting Methods – Similarities and Differences
Developing a Working Model

Tony Wigram

Introduction and overview

Songwriting is a frequently and flexibly used method of intervention in music therapy. The chapters in this book describe and define an impressive range of methods, and demonstrate how they are applied to specific populations. The authors of these chapters have demonstrated some important consistency in their approaches, as well as in the stages of song creation that they have reported. The intention and focus of this book was to report therapists' methods and clinical techniques in utilizing songwriting in therapy, with relevant clinical vignettes or examples to illustrate the method. It is intended as a methods book – with the expectation that readers can see and learn from an explanation of the staged process of songwriting how it can be applied in therapy (and why), and that the procedures for any specific techniques that have been developed and applied are clearly described. For clinicians, educators and students, the book is partly intended as a 'tutor' where an understanding of, and the technical requirements for, the application of songwriting can be learnt, and specific techniques used in its application to different populations can also be differentiated.

The way in which authors explain their methods varies considerably, even if the underlying methods are similar. The style of presentations has included:

- explanation of method followed by case examples
- explanation of method with case vignettes included at each stage as examples
- description of process mainly based on clinical examples that refer to method.

The majority of chapters have explained the method of songwriting in therapy from the perspective of the creation of a song, and its value as an outcome of a therapeutic process. Two chapters differ from this, one (Oldfield and Franke) because this was concerned with a process of spontaneous and improvised song creation without a staged development of the product, and the other (Krout) because the song was created by the therapist for the group.

Reference to theory

The authors contributing to this book have come from a wide variety of therapeutic orientations and culturally diverse backgrounds. There are those trained in the more humanistic/analytical approaches of the European music therapy tradition, others from the more cognitive and behavioural orientation of the US, and the authors from Australia who, I think it can be said, are often balancing the structured, behaviourally oriented approach with the humanistic influences to which they are also exposed. Despite this, there is not a heavy weighting in the contributions on the theoretical framework within which any of the authors' songwriting approaches may be centred. The influences of therapeutic orientation tend to emerge more in the description of clinical examples, and in particular from the therapist's commentary on the value of songwriting for a particular client, than in the methods or techniques used.

Definition

In the opening chapter, Wigram and Baker offered a provisional definition of songwriting in music therapy as:

> The process of creating, notating and/or recording lyrics and music by the client or clients and therapist within a therapeutic relationship to address psychosocial, emotional, cognitive and communication needs of the client.

Considering the authors have presented a range and variety of models, methods and techniques, the majority still meet the general criteria of this definition. Perhaps the model that does not really match is where the therapist and client are simultaneously and spontaneously improvising a song that is therefore created in the here and now, and is not intended to be 'constructed' in the traditional sense, refined, and written down in any form and recorded.

It is important at this stage to clarify what is meant by 'method' and what is meant by 'technique'. Therapeutic methods are the approaches chosen by the therapist to achieve therapeutic change and can be understood as the 'method' of work. Conversely, techniques are the tools and strategies, musical activities and concrete therapist-initiated musical experiences which are integral to the success of the applied method. There are many examples of therapists who have developed

Table 12.1 Structure or flexibility in songwriting approaches

Chapter	Author(s)	Population	Type of protocol
1	Oldfield and Franke	Children	Improvised song creation; flexible with a basic 'story-building' structure
2	Davies	Child psychiatry	Broad structure involving guiding principles for improvised and structured songwriting
3	Derrington	Adolescents	Structured and semi-structured: 10-stage structured model; 4-stage semi-structured model
4	Day	Adults abused in childhood	Group approach; 4-step, structured approach
5	Rolvsjord	Adult psychiatry	Broad guidelines on lyric and melody creation
6	Baker *et al.*	Children and adults with traumatic brain injury	Structured approach in stages for lyrics and music; techniques for music composition
7	Baker	Adults with traumatic brain injury	Structured approach in stages for lyrics; techniques for music composition
8	Aasgaard	Child oncology	Guiding principles based on issues for children with cancer
9	O'Brien	Adult oncology	5-stage semi-structured method
10	Krout	Bereaved teenagers	10-step structure
11	Dileo and Magill	Adult oncology and hospice	Multicultural model; semi-structured methods used

protocols, procedures and method in their approach to using songwriting, and other examples where the improvised nature of the process has required a much freer and less defined protocol. The types of protocol used by each author, with reference to the degree of structure described, are listed in Table 12.1.

Relevance to different populations

Songwriting in music therapy will have different therapeutic objectives depending on the needs and expectations of the individual or group with whom the method is being applied. There is an evident diversity and clinical relevance to the rationale behind the use of songwriting in therapy, with most therapists employing this method referring to its value as a vehicle for expression of feelings. There are many other clinically specific reasons, ranging from pragmatic skill development (Baker) to management of pain (Dileo and Magill). Nevertheless, a majority find that the creation of songs provides a tool for externalizing emotions, and consequently the themes listed in Table 12.2 often relate to the client's emotional life, and the issues, experiences and conflicts with which they have been, are or expect to be working in therapy.

The range of themes and, more specifically, the nature of these themes in relation to the various populations and their therapeutic needs require appropriate and sometimes flexible working tools – and methods – for their application to the medium of songs. It is evident that therapists reporting on songwriting are sensitive not only to the needs of the clients, but also to the importance of the client's need to value the song as something with which they themselves have collaborated in creating, if not completely composed by themselves. This requires particular skills in both lyric construction and, more importantly, music composition when a majority of clients will often have never before tried to compose a song. In fact, while the separate arts of writing poetry and verse and composing melody and harmony can be sophisticated, complex and challenging, the therapists who report their method of engaging clients in songwriting demonstrate very well how, with a wide variety of clearly thought-out strategies and techniques, they have developed a number of procedures that enable and empower clients to overcome (or avoid) complexity, and achieve their goal.

It is not surprising, given this ability, that many therapists report the nurturing and development of self-esteem as one of the therapeutic outcomes. Almost everyone could have a dream that they would write a satisfying and satisfactory song, perhaps in the same way that we could dream about writing a successful novel, or painting a fine picture. It is within the grasp of all human beings to be able to represent something in an art media, and as songs have such a wide appeal in everyday life, this is a dream to which all could aspire. Therefore, the methods by which therapists facilitate songwriting are of particular interest. In the next section, protocols, lyric creation and music creation used in songwriting will all be reviewed, with a list of commonly used methods presented at the end.

Table 12.2 Themes of songs relevant to the population defined in the chapter

Chapter	Author(s)	Population	Themes
1	Oldfield and Franke	Children	'Once upon a time...' themes: animals; people; fairy tales
2	Davies	Child psychiatry	Musical themes; relating to others
3	Derrington	Adolescents	Youth culture; relationships; emotions; violence; negative feelings
4	Day	Adults abused in childhood	Effects of abuse; self-esteem; anger; trust; domestic violence; social isolation; verbal abuse; communication; self-harm; body image; suicide; stress; relaxation
5	Rolvsjord	Adult psychiatry	Clients' experiences, emotions and issues
6	Baker *et al.*	Children and adults with traumatic brain injury	Adjusting to trauma and change; distress; pain; hospitalization; dependency; helplessness; anger
7	Baker	Adults with traumatic brain injury	Self-reflection; relationships; events; concrete daily topics (i.e. weather)
8	Aasgaard	Child oncology	Hospitalization; medical procedures; emotional expression/feeling; achievement; relationships; humour
9	O'Brien	Adult oncology	Past, present and future; hopes and dreams; relationships; family; dying
10	Krout	Bereaved teenagers	Expression of feelings; processing grief; empowerment
11	Dileo and Magill	Adult oncology and hospice	Family-related issues; closure; resolution; emotional expression; facing death

Characteristics of methods of songwriting

Most authors reporting on the use of songwriting as a tool in music therapy in the literature centre their writing on case reports with occasional or implicit reference to method. In this book, authors have reported in detail on the methods they use, and in broad terms they have described their procedure, the method of developing the lyrics and the music for a song, the therapeutic value of the process, what happens to a song and its ongoing role in a person's life.

Protocols and procedures

There is a wide spectrum in terms of the defined protocols authors have reported, with descriptions of the way the therapists work ranging from quite structured approaches with pre-defined steps or stages, to more spontaneous, free styles of work. Table 12.3 gives an overview of differing methods.

Table 12.3 Types of structured, semi-structured or improvised protocols

Chapter	Author(s)	Population	Type of protocol
1	Oldfield and Franke	Children	Story-making structure with improvised 'sound effects'; therapist-led initially, incorporating child's ideas
2	Davies	Child psychiatry	Broad structure: brainstorming a theme; creating lyrics; composing the music; performing and recording
3	Derrington	Adolescents	Stages involving: developing themes; finding and writing lyrics; choosing musical style; creating music; scoring; recording
4	Day	Adults abused in childhood	4-step, structured approach involving: brainstorming themes; lyric creation; music creation; rehearsing/recording
5	Rolvsjord	Adult psychiatry	No specific procedure; co-creation of lyrics; therapist creation of melody or improvised by therapist and client
6	Baker *et al.*	Children and adults with traumatic brain injury	Structured approach: therapeutic lyric creation; techniques of musical composition or adaption

Continued on next page

Table 12.3 (cont.)

Chapter	Author(s)	Population	Type of protocol
7	Baker	Adults with traumatic brain injury	Structured approach: therapeutic lyric creation; techniques of musical composition or adaption
8	Aasgaard	Child oncology	A loose procedure: promoting interest; developing lyrics; sound/rhythm/melody; accompaniment; different versions of the song; performing; recording
9	O'Brien	Adult oncology	Guiding Original Lyrics and Music (GOLM) – a 5-stage process involving: brainstorming; structural reframing; style and key; melody and accompaniment; presenting and recording
10	Krout	Bereaved teenagers	10-step protocol: who is writing and purpose; lyrics or music; rough lyrics; style; design lyrics; develop harmony; develop melody; create verse–chorus; add stylistic features
11	Dileo and Magill	Adult oncology and hospice	Culturally familiar song forms are used; variable protocols

Lyric creation techniques

The creation of lyrics is a common starting point for songwriting in therapy, where the model used with verbal clients has the intention of constructing and composing a 'new' song. As defined in Table 12.4, there are two clear aspects to the creation of lyrics described by all of the authors, the method of lyric composition and the style of lyrics (or poetry) used.

There are two exceptions where the creation of lyrics does not precede the composition of music. First, when the therapist or client is using existing songs where they write up new, relevant lyrics to the existing music of songs they like. The other model is where the music emerges in an improvised way simultaneously with the lyrics, or where a story is being developed with an improvised musical accompaniment.

There is also an interesting range of techniques for the development of lyrics, which range from pre-composed by either client or therapist and brought to the session, to an example of free association where words are spontaneously generated from the client related to the experiences they are undergoing in treatment, and then identified as themes.

Table 12.4 Lyric creation techniques specified in the chapter

Chapter	Author(s)	Population	Method of lyric composition	Lyric style used
1	Oldfield and Franke	Children	Improvised; therapist introduces story theme	Free; story building
2	Davies	Child psychiatry	Pre-composed by children at home; therapist writes down and may offer structure	Verse and chorus; free verse
3	Derrington	Adolescents	Clients bring pre-composed lyrics/poetry: lyrics drawn from existing songs; spontaneous in session	Verse and chorus; rhyme; phrasing
4	Day	Adults abused in childhood	Identify key issues; discuss issues; identify main idea; write lyrics 'Homework' by group members	Verse and repeated chorus model
5	Rolvsjord	Adult psychiatry	Co-creation: selecting words from list; self-generated; client's poem	Verse and chorus style
6	Baker et al.	Children and adults with traumatic brain injury	Therapeutic lyric creation – 9 stages: finding topics; selecting; brainstorming ideas; identify principal idea; developing idea; grouping ideas; discard irrelevant ideas; construct outline; write lyrics	Existing songs; verse and chorus style; free verse; rhyming verse
7	Baker	Adults with traumatic brain injury	Therapeutic lyric creation – 9 stages: finding topics; selecting; brainstorming ideas; identify principal idea; developing idea; grouping ideas; discard irrelevant ideas; construct outline; write lyrics	Existing songs; verse and chorus style; free verse; rhyming verse
8	Aasgaard	Child oncology	Child chooses words, subjects, themes or a text	Rhyming style; free style verse
9	O'Brien	Adult oncology	Patients and therapist brainstorm ideas; structural reframing of ideas; lyric creation	Verse, chorus, bridge, refrain
10	Krout	Bereaved teenagers	Therapist develops lyrics based on grief-related themes; strategic songwriting (Brunk 1998)	Verse–chorus style
11	Dileo and Magill	Adult oncology and hospice	Clients suggest themes from which lyrics can be created	Variable – depending on cultural style

Music creation techniques

There are clear differences in how therapists go about the process of creating the music to the lyrics. Some use instruments, some begin with an accompaniment pattern, while others offer possible musical elements and styles to the client, concerned that, from the very beginning, the style of music in the song will be very much the decision of the client and, as much as possible, the construction of the client. Table 12.5 presents an overview of these different methods of music creation reported by therapists working with songwriting.

What happens to the created song during the therapy process, or when therapy finishes? Is there a therapeutic goal for the song to be other than a product of the client, owned by the client, and subsequently used by the client alone? Again, there is some diversity in the final functions of songs in therapy.

Table 12.5 Music creation techniques specified in the chapter

Chapter	Author(s)	Population	Method of musical composition	Different song styles reported as used
1	Oldfield and Franke	Children	Improvised; child with pitched and un-pitched percussion; tonal harmonic structures	'Choir boy'; singing; rock; rap; pop; opera
2	Davies	Child psychiatry	Using material from known songs; improvising	Material from preferred songs and pieces
3	Derrington	Adolescents	Students jam; improvising musical effects; drawing on material from pop songs	Using material from pop songs; mobile phone tunes; simple tonal harmonies; boogie-woogie
4	Day	Adults abused in childhood	Decision steps: melody and accompaniment style; genre; instrumentation; song style; group decision	Variable – no pre-conceived style
5	Rolvsjord	Adult psychiatry	Therapist creates melody and harmony or therapist and client improvise melodies over simple harmonic base	Norwegian folk; popular music style 2-chord/4-chord pattern; uses Austin (2002) vocal holding

Continued on next page

Table 12.5 (cont.)

Chapter	Author(s)	Population	Method of musical composition	Different song styles reported as used
6	Baker *et al.*	Children and adults with traumatic brain injury	Use of existing songs: fill-in-the-blank; song parody; song collage; composed	Existing songs; popular music: rhythm and blues; heavy metal; hip hop; Euro-pop
7	Baker	Adults with traumatic brain injury	Use of existing songs: fill-in-the-blank; song parody; song collage; composed	Popular music: rhythm and blues; heavy metal; hip hop; Euro-pop
8	Aasgaard	Child oncology	Existing songs (song parody); therapist created	Children's songs; popular songs
9	O'Brien	Adult oncology	Creating with the patient: the GOLM method involves constructing the song in short sections, confirming style, key, melody, harmony, accompaniment, lyric setting	Pop; jazz; funk; rock; country; grunge; techno; folk; classical; ballads; blues; R&B; soul; gospel; trad; nonsense; rap; ambient pop; alternative
10	Krout	Bereaved teenagers	Created by the therapist for the clients as exemplified in this chapter	Uses stylistic options including: folk, blues, jazz, contemporary, alternative, classical, show-songs
11	Dileo and Magill	Adult oncology and hospice	Created by the therapist with culturally appropriate styles for clients	Culturally familiar song forms are used, e.g. Latino; Klezmer Doina; African; African American; Eastern Indian

Authors have made reference to the therapeutic relevance of the song for clients, and in what way they might become a final 'object' – a recorded song. Table 12.6 illustrates the spectrum of the different 'lives' songs may have for each of the populations reported, as well as summarizing the therapeutic values authors have identified to the process.

For some, the created songs were evidently of an intensely private and confidential nature, and they were not either recorded or performed. The material that may be contained in the lyrics could represent personal anguish, fear, anxiety, pain and

Table 12.6 The extended life and function of created songs

Chapter	Author(s)	Population	Relevance of song in therapy	The final product
1	Oldfield and Franke	Children	Externalize childhood thoughts, fantasies, emotions, conflicts in the improvised song; for diagnosis	As improvised material the final product may or may not be recorded
2	Davies	Child psychiatry	For self-esteem; self-confidence; uncovering talent; achievement; validating experiences	Variable: the song can stay in the music therapy room, or go beyond
3	Derrington	Adolescents	Development of identity; self-expression; addressing anxiety and behavioural problems	Recording; saving in song folders; improvised
4	Day	Adults abused in childhood	Processing painful memories and experiences; the expression and validation of feelings within a group context; empowerment; trust	Rehearsing and recording the song onto a CD is of major importance for this population
5	Rolvsjord	Adult psychiatry	Resource orientated: identity building; amplifying strengths; working on competencies of client	Not specified
6	Baker et al.	Children and adults with traumatic brain injury	Identifying and externalizing emotions; communicating to loved ones; self-motivation and encouragement; simply telling their story	Audio recording and transcribed version (lyrics only) provided to patient
7	Baker	Adults with traumatic brain injury	Pragmatic skill redevelopment; functional skills; redeveloping conversation skills; initiating and developing topics	Audio recording and transcribed version (lyrics only) provided to patient; song folder; home and family pictures included for child clients

Continued on next page

Table 12.6 (cont.)

Chapter	Author(s)	Population	Relevance of song in therapy	The final product
8	Aasgaard	Child oncology	To normalize, brighten the environment; as a work of art; social experience; externalizing distress and pain	Audio recordings; making CDs; the songs become part of life beyond hospital – school, home
9	O'Brien	Adult oncology	Positive pleasurable experience; personal record; help clarify thinking; calming; self-expression; self-esteem; quality of life	Written text; audio recordings; professional CD recordings
10	Krout	Bereaved teenagers	For discussion and verbal processing, as well as for related arts activities such as drawing, painting, poetry, collage making and movement	Mainly for the group setting; one 'presentation' of a song in a larger group context with other clients addressing similar issues
11	Dileo and Magill	Adult oncology and hospice	Self-expression; enhancement of spirituality; life review; relationship closure; management of pain; regularize breathing	Variable: songs are sometimes recorded for playing to children and relatives

misery, and the song becomes a therapeutic container for such feelings and emotions. While taking this into consideration, it is nevertheless true that song-writing as a method in music therapy can provide a tangible artistic outcome, in the form of a written song. This is a method in music therapy that is closest to art therapy, where the client (and therapist) amass a portfolio of material, be it drawings, paintings or sculptures, which represent a therapeutic journey over time. It is a tangible product, by which a client can see from where he has come, and where he is. While not referring to this specifically, some therapists using songwriting neverthe-less refer to changing material in songs over time. The lyrics are perhaps most likely to represent this therapeutic change, although not exclusively. Music also holds an important role in supporting or defining the mood or emotional content of songs.

Commonly reported methods and techniques

The most important contribution made by many authors writing on the subject of songwriting in music therapy is to define and describe specific methods in writing the songs. For anyone who would like to begin to incorporate this method of work into their clinical practice, and for the training of therapists, a description of the specific methods used is essential in developing therapeutic applications. The following lists of reported techniques of lyric creation and music creation are drawn from this literature.

Techniques of lyric creation in songwriting

Therapeutic lyric creation (Baker; O'Callaghan 1996) A 9-stage structured approach to creating the lyrics of a song before the music is developed.

Guiding free brainstorming (O'Brien) A patient is encouraged to speak freely about any topic, while the therapist transcribes words and then draws out salient comments or remarks.

Guiding Original Lyrics and Music (GOLM) (O'Brien) A 5-step process guiding the patient through songwriting, developing lyrics and offering musical examples from which to choose.

Selecting words from a list of words (Rolvsjord) A list of words and symbols can be created from stories the clients have shared and from songs client and therapist have sung or listened to within the therapy sessions.

Client self-generates words (Rolvsjord) Client spontaneously generates some words which the therapist formulates into song using open or poetic structure.

Client writes a poem (Rolvsjord; Derrington) Sometimes clients contribute their material in the form of a poem. In these situations, the exact wording in the poem is not always identical with the lyrics in the final product of the song.

Role playing and acting out (Derrington) Clients can use play equipment such as puppets, pretend mobile phones, art materials, etc., creatively to generate themes and lyrics.

Fill-in-the-Blank Technique (FBT) (Baker; Baker *et al.*; Aasgaard) A technique using a familiar song may be adopted. A song that the client relates to may be used and adapted to make it more personally relevant. This technique provides more structure for clients who may have difficulty expanding and organizing simple ideas, and can also provide direction for the lyrics and may serve as a beginning point for a client who is having trouble getting started.

Song Parody Technique (SPT) (Aasgaard; Baker; Baker *et al.*; Dileo and Magill) Uses the music of a pre-composed song whereby the lyrics of the original song are completely replaced by client-generated lyrics. In many cases a combination of the SPT and FBT is employed.

Song Collage Technique (SCT) (Baker; Baker *et al.*) Another technique, which can be helpful for clients who have difficulty identifying or articulating their emotions, is the use of 'song collage'. This technique involves the client looking through music books or the lyric sheet within CD covers and selecting words or phrases from pre-composed songs that stand out, or have personal significance to them.

Use of Rhyme Technique (URT) (Baker; Baker *et al.*) The use of rhyming lyric patterns can be employed to create structure in a song. If a client is able to generate lists of words that rhyme with key words that they have included, then this technique is a good way to expand and organize song ideas.

Use of lyrics from existing songs (Derrington) The clients draw on lyrics from already composed songs.

Pre-composed poems/lyrics/verse (Derrington) The clients bring a poem, verse or lyric they have composed previously in another situation.

Home-based lyric development (Day) Clients work on lyrics through jotting down ideas or images in between sessions

Spontaneous structured story making (Oldfield and Franke) Starting with a therapist-led 'Once upon a time...' opening, the client and therapist build up an improvised story.

Constructing the song in sections (O'Brien) Breaking down the songwriting process into sections of the song, which reduces the possibility of the creative process as a whole appearing too daunting for the patient.

Externalizing internal aspects of self (Oldfield and Franke) Storytelling methods that draw out clients' thoughts and feelings, self-reflections and unconscious material.

Therapist–scribe (Davies) Therapists act as the 'scribe' to write down the spontaneously created words and phrases of the client(s), and may help structure them into usable lyrics.

Open-ended questions (O'Brien) Used to gather more general information about a theme; for example, 'You mentioned you had many dreams for your future. Could you tell me more about this?'

Direct questions (O'Brien) Used when trying to obtain more detail from the patient to clarify themes; for example, 'Do these hopes and dreams sustain you during this time?'

Yes, no, or choice questions (O'Brien) Used when guiding the patient towards making a decision about his or her theme, for example, 'Would you like your song to focus on your future or your past?'

Structural reframing (O'Brien) Used for directing the free brainstorming towards a song structure, encouraging the patient to think of his/her material in terms of song structure such as the chorus, verse/s and other sections of the song. Draws together the patient's themes and words from the transcription. Groups ideas into a song structure.

Validation, identification, normalization and expression (*VINE*) (Krout) A general on-going counselling for bereaved emotions and teenagers utilized by Krout in songwriting for the expression of feelings, thoughts and emotions.

Strategic songwriting (Brunk 1998) The process of composing a song ahead of time for a specific goal and/or client.

Techniques of music creation in songwriting

Improvisation (Oldfield and Franke) Using instruments and therapist supported improvised music-making while spontaneously creating a song.

Music sound effects (Oldfield and Franke) Instruments used to improvise sound effects to story or developing lyrics.

Word painting (Davies; O'Brien) Creating music that represents or describes the emotion or image of a word or phrase.

Using pre-composed melodies or parts of melodies (Derrington) Clients choose to use melodies and parts of melodies from existing songs to inspire or structure their musical composition.

Therapist-created–client-accepted decision process (Day) Where the client(s) clearly identify the therapist as 'responsible' for the music creation, the therapist offers musical elements and places the client(s) in the position of deciding what the music could be like.

Improvised melody over 2-chord/4-chord pattern (Rolvsjord; Austin 1999, 2002) Using a simple 2- or 4-chord harmonic pattern to create an atmosphere appropriate to the theme communicated within the lyrics. A warm-up exercise to become familiar with the harmonic scheme is followed by improvising a melody, taking turns in singing every second phrase.

Determining the style and key of the song (O'Brien) Offering the patient different styles and asking the patient about his or her preferred genre of music for the song.

Spontaneously underpinning the melody (O'Brien) Encouraging the patient to actively choose chord progressions where the harmonic framework will provide a relevant context for setting the lyrics to an appropriate 'musical' mood.

Setting the melody and accompaniment: secondary reframing (O'Brien) Once the music style is selected, further changes to the lyrics may need to be made to align with the style.

Notating the music in a session (O'Brien) Using a type of melodic shorthand to cue the therapist's musical memory of the song when notating melodies, and also when notating the chords of an accompaniment or harmonic frame.

Collectivist (African-American, Asian, Hispanic) (Dileo and Magill) Songs involving the participation of more than one person; songs involving improvised dialogues between or among two or more participants; songs providing the vehicle for intense expression of emotion; songs where egalitarian relationships are emphasized; call and response structures are common.

Song narratives (Dileo and Magill) The lyrics are 'sung' within a very limited melodic range, on one pitch, or in rhythmic chant form. Specifically, the lyrics are performed in a type of 'spoken song' (*Sprechgesang*), a musical style that may appear more accessible to a medically frail patient. These lyrics can be supported by a chordal harmonic progression. The song structure may be strophic or through-composed, and a repetitive refrain may be employed to emphasize specific content, for example an over-arching meaning, event or person.

A flexible, generic working model

There are many variations on a basic model that can be seen in a majority of chapters. With the exception of Oldfield and Franke, and Krout, where the songs used were either purely emerging from spontaneous, 'here and now' improvisation, or as a pre-composed song created for a group or individual, the generic model involves a sequence of logical and predictable stages, where the variability tends to be found in who takes the initiative or responsibility for developing the lyrics and music. Some authors refer to *steps* in the process while others describe *stages*. There is some difference in my perception between these two terms, where *stages* refer to a more time oriented phase of the activity, while *steps* tends to indicate a procedural, possibly hierarchical, level which relates to something that is achieved before moving up to the next step.

The working model I am presenting below describes the process with stages rather than steps, and offers a number of methods, one or more of which can be used depending on the client population to which the method is being applied. It should be considered as a guidance structure and used in conjunction with both the range of lyric creation techniques and music creation techniques listed above, as well as with reference to the clinically specific approaches described by many authors experienced in using songs in therapy.

Flexible Approach to Songwriting in Therapy (FAST)

STAGE 1: INTRODUCTION TO SONGWRITING

- Method 1   Improvising incorporating story creation
- Method 2   Therapist proposes idea in discussion
- Method 3   Client requests idea following song singing

STAGE 2: FORMULATION OF LYRICS

- Method 1   Brainstorming themes (client and therapist)
- Method 2   Words are spontaneously suggested (client or therapist)
- Method 3   Words relating to client issues suggested (client or therapist)
- Method 4   Client brings pre-composed lyrics

STAGE 3: DEVELOPMENT OF MUSIC

- Method 1   Improvised (client and therapist)
- Method 2   Improvised melody over structured harmonic frame (client and/or therapist)
- Method 3   Clients create melody and harmony
- Method 4   Therapist offers ideas in short fragments or chords of melody and harmony, accepted or rejected by client
- Method 5   Therapist creates music to client's lyrics

STAGE 4: WRITING DOWN A SONG

- Method 1   Lyrics only
- Method 2   Lyrics and melody
- Method 3   Lyrics, melody and basic guitar/piano chordal harmonic structure
- Method 4   Lyrics, melody, harmony and accompaniment – full version

STAGE 5: PERFORMING OF SONG[1]

- Method 1   The song is performed by client and therapist together
- Method 2   The song is performed to staff and other clients
- Method 3   The song is performed to family and friends

STAGE 6: RECORDING OF SONG

- Method 1   The song is recorded by client and therapist in an original form
- Method 2   Group work – group recording
- Method 3   Music transcribed and orchestrated for professional recording

This model is intended to provide an adaptable framework, where the therapist (or client) can deploy the most relevant, appropriate and therapeutically fruitful method during each stage of the process. The methods were described with the intention that they could be suitable for all age ranges, while still having discrete characteristics that would differentiate them to population and pathology.

Conclusion

I return to the position stated in the introduction chapter of this book, 'Music began with singing' (Sachs 1969, p.4). The therapists who have contributed to this text are a sample from a still quite small group of music therapists worldwide who have

---

1   Stages 5 and 6 are interchangeable.

applied the method of songwriting in therapy. There is no doubt that there are specialized skills in songwriting. It is interesting that only limited attention is paid to teaching these methods to therapists during their basic training and there are no advanced courses offered in these techniques. Much time is devoted to developing song singing skills, music-making skills and improvisation skills. It was the intention of this book, as with a previous book (Wigram 2004), to write as clearly and comprehensively as possible about the methods and techniques used, in order that this method of therapy, to date quite significantly underdeveloped, can be more widely and appropriately applied. Songs always will be a natural container for the thoughts, feelings, emotions, personality characteristics, dreams and fantasies of people from all age ranges and, as such, provide a natural musical medium for the therapeutic process.

References

Aasgaard, T. (2000) 'A suspiciously cheerful lady: a study of a song's life in the paediatric oncology ward and beyond.' *British Journal of Music Therapy 14*, 70–82.

Aasgaard, T. (2001) 'An ecology of love: aspects of music therapy in the paediatric oncology environment.' *Journal of Palliative Care 17*, 3, 177–183.

Aasgaard, T. (2002) 'Song creations by children with cancer: process and meaning.' Unpublished PhD thesis, Institute for Music and Music Therapy, Aalborg University.

Aasgaard, T. (2004a) 'A Pied Piper among white coats and infusion pumps.' In G. Ansdell and M. Pavlicevic (eds) *Community Music Therapy – International Initiatives*. London: Jessica Kingsley Publishers.

Aasgaard, T. (2004b) 'Song creations by children with cancer: process and meaning.' In D. Aldridge (ed) *Case Study Designs in Music Therapy*. London: Jessica Kingsley Publishers.

Abad, V. (2003) 'A time of turmoil: music therapy interventions for adolescents in a paediatric oncology ward.' *Australian Journal of Music Therapy 14*, 20–37.

Abidin, R. (1995) *Parenting Stress Index*. Third edition. Odessa, FL: Psychological Assessment Resources.

Adams, C. (2002) 'Practitioner review: the assessment of language pragmatics.' *Journal of Psychology and Psychiatry 43*, 8, 973–987.

Aigen, K. (2004) 'Conversations on creating community: performance as music therapy in New York city.' In M. Pavlicevic and G. Ansdell (eds) *Community Music Therapy*. London: Jessica Kingsley Publishers.

Alexander, D.A. (1993) 'Psychological/social research.' In D. Doyle, G.W.C. Hanks and N. Macdonald (eds) *Oxford Textbook of Palliative Medicine*. Oxford: Oxford University Press.

Austin, D. (1999) 'Vocal improvisation in analytically oriented music therapy with adults.' In T. Wigram and J. De Backer (eds) *Clinical Applications of Music Therapy in Psychiatry*. London: Jessica Kingsley Publishers.

Austin, D. (2002) 'The voice of trauma: a wounded healer's perspective.' In J. Sutton (ed) *Music, Music Therapy and Trauma*. London: Jessica Kingsley Publishers.

Bailey, L.M. (1984) 'The use of songs in music therapy with cancer patients and their families.' *Music Therapy 4*, 1, 5–17.

Baker, F., Kennelly, J. and Tamplin, J. (in press[a]) 'Themes in song writing by clients with TBI: Differences across the lifespan.' *Australian Journal of Music Therapy*.

Baker, F., Kennelly, J. and Tamplin, J. (in press[b]) 'Adjustment to traumatic brain injury through song writing: reviewing the past and looking to the future.' *Brain Impairment*.

Baker, F., Kennelly, J. and Tamplin, J. (in press[c]) 'Themes in song writing by clients with TBI: gender differences.' *Journal of Music Therapy*.

Bass, E. and Davis, L. (1988) *The Courage to Heal: A Guide for Women Survivors of Child Sexual Abuse*. New York: Harper and Row.

Biddle, K.R., McCabe, A. and Bliss, L.S. (1996) 'Narrative skills following traumatic brain injury in children and adults.' *Journal of Communication Disorders 29*, 447–469.

Blume, J. (2004) *Six Steps to Songwriting Success*. New York: Billboard Books.

Borod, J.C., Pick, L.H., Andelman, F., Obler, L.K., Welkowitz, J., Rorie, K.D., Bloom, R.L., Campbell, A.L., Tweedy, J.R. and Sliwinski, M. (2000) 'Verbal pragmatics following unilateral stroke: emotional content and valence.' *Neuropsychology 14*, 1, 112–124.

Bright, R. (2002) *Supportive Eclectic Music Therapy for Grief and Loss*. St Louis: MMB Music.

Brunk, B.K. (1998) *Songwriting for Music Therapists*. Grapevine, TX: Prelude Music Therapy.

Bruscia, K. (1987) *Improvisational Models of Music Therapy*. Springfield, IL: Charles C. Thomas.

Bruscia, K. (1998) *The Dynamics of Music Psychotherapy*. Phoenixville: Barcelona Publishers.

Burns, S., Harbuz, M., Hucklebridge, F. and Bunt, L. (2001) 'A pilot study into the therapeutic effects of music therapy at a cancer help center.' *Alternative Therapy and Health Medicine 7*, 48–56.

Carter, E. (2004) 'Thank you for the music: an exploration of music therapy for a child with severe psychosomatic symptoms.' Paper presented at the *Sixth European Music Therapy Conference*, Jyväskylä, Finland.

Cassileth, B., Vickers, A. and Magill, L. (2003) 'Music therapy for mood disturbance during hospitalization for autologous stem cell transplantation: a randomized controlled trial.' *Cancer 98*, 2723–2729. DOI: 10.1002/cncr.11842.

Charmaz, K. (1995) 'The body, identity, and self: adapting to impairments.' *Sociological Quarterly 36*, 657–680.

Clendenon-Wallen, J. (1991) 'The use of music therapy to influence the self-confidence and self-esteem of adolescents who are sexually abused.' *Music Therapy Perspectives 9*, 73–81.

Coates, A., Abraham, S., Kaye, S.B., Sowerbutts, T., Frewin, C., Fox, R.M. and Tattersall, M.H.N. (1983) 'On the receiving end – patient perception of side-effects of cancer chemotherapy.' *European Journal of Cancer and Clinical Oncology 19*, 203–208.

Cordobés, T.K. (1997) 'Group songwriting as a method of developing group cohesion for HIV-seropositive adult patients with depression.' *Journal of Music Therapy 34*, 1, 46–67.

Cosby, B. (1988) *Fatherhood*. Garden City, New York: Guild Publishing.

Courtois, C.A. (1988) *Healing the Incest Wound: Adult Survivors in Therapy*. New York: Norton.

Dalton, T. (1999) 'The use of songwriting in working with children in bereavement.' Paper presented at the Fall Continuing Education Workshops of the Florida Association for Music Therapy: *Music Therapy in Hospice and Palliative Care*, West Palm Beach, Florida.

Dalton, T. (2002) 'Songwriting: a music therapy intervention with bereaved adolescents.' Presented at the Music Therapy for Bereavement Symposium of the Florida Association for Music Therapy, *Hospice of the Comforter*, Altamonte Springs, Florida.

Dalton, T.A. and Krout, R.E. (2005) 'Development of the Grief Process Scale through music therapy songwriting with bereaved adolescents.' *The Arts in Psychotherapy, 32* (2), 131–143.

Davis, W.B., Gfeller, K.E. and Thaut, M.H. (1999) *An Introduction to Music Therapy: Theory and Practice*. Second edition. Boston, MA: McGraw-Hill.

De Backer, J. (1993) 'Containment in music therapy.' In M. Heal and T. Wigram (eds) *Music Therapy in Health and Education*. London: Jessica Kingsley Publishers.

DeNora, T. (2000) *Music in Everyday Life*. Cambridge: Cambridge University Press.

DeNora, T. (2003) *After Adorno: Rethinking Music Sociology*. Cambridge: Cambridge University Press.

Dilavore, P., Rutter, M. and Lord, C. (1995) 'The prelinguistic autistic diagnostic schedule.' *Journal of Autism and Developmental Disorders 25*, 4, 355–379.

Dileo, C. (2000) *Ethical Thinking in Music Therapy*. Cherry Hill, NJ: Jeffrey Books.

Dileo, C. and Parker, C. (2005) 'Songs at the end of life.' In C. Dileo and J. Loewy (eds) *Music Therapy at the End of Life*. Cherry Hill, NJ: Jeffrey Books.

Dowland, J. (1600) 'Flow, my tears.' Strophic song for lute.

Duncan, B.L. and Miller, S.D. (2000) *The Heroic Client: Doing Client-Directed, Outcome-Informed Therapy*. San Francisco: Jossey-Bass and Wiley Co.

Edgerton, C.D. (1990) 'Creative group songwriting.' *Music Therapy Perspectives 8*, 15–19.

Edwards, J. (1998) 'Music therapy for children with severe burn injury.' *Music Therapy Perspectives 16*, 21–26.

Eriksson, E.H. (1963) *Childhood and Society*. Second edition. New York: Norton.

Eriksson, E.H. (1968) *Identity, Youth and Crisis*. New York: Norton.

Ezzone, S., Baker, C., Rosselet, R. and Terepka, E. (1998) 'Music as an adjunct to antiemetic therapy.' *Oncology Nursing Forum 25*, 1551–1556.

Fenton, M. and Hughes, P. (1989) *Passivity to Empowerment*. London: Royal Association for Disability and Rehabilitation.

Ficken, T. (1976) 'The use of songwriting in a psychiatric setting.' *Journal of Music Therapy 13*, 4, 163–172.

Fischer, R. (1991) 'Original song drawings in the treatment of a developmental disabled, autistic young man.' In K. Bruscia (ed) *Case Studies in Music Therapy*. Pheonixville: Barcelona Publishers.

Flower, C. (1993) 'Control and creativity: music therapy with adolescents in secure care.' In M. Heal and T. Wigram (eds) *Music Therapy in Health and Education*. London: Jessica Kingsley Publishers.

Foy, D., Eriksson, C. and Trice, G. (2001) 'Introduction to group interventions for trauma survivors.' *Group Dynamics, Theory, Research and Practice 5*, 4, 246–251.

Freed, B.S. (1987) 'Songwriting with the chemically dependent.' *Music Therapy Perspectives 4*, 13–18.

Gass, R. and Brehony, K. (1999) *Chanting: Discovering the Spirit in Sound*. New York: Broadway Books.

Gfeller, K. (1987) 'Songwriting as a tool for reading and language remediation.' *Music Therapy 6*, 2, 28–38.

Gillette, S. (1995) *Songwriting and the Creative Process*. Bethlehem, PA: Sing Out.

Glassman, L.R. (1991) 'Music therapy and bibliotherapy in the rehabilitation of traumatic brain injury: a case study.' *The Arts in Psychotherapy 18*, 149–156.

Goldstein, S.L. (1990) 'A songwriting assessment for hopelessness in depressed adolescents: a review of the literature and a pilot study.' *Arts in Psychotherapy 17*, 117–124.

Grice, H.P. (1978) 'Further notes on logic and conversation.' In P. Cole (ed) *Syntax and Semantics: Pragmatics*. New York: Academic Press.

Griessmeier, B. and Bossinger, W. (1994) *Musiktherapie mit Krebskranken Kindern*. Stuttgart: Gustav Fisscher Verlag.

Grønnesby, J.P. (2004) *...om håp, savn og kjærlighet: 11 sanger (...on hope, privation and love: 11 songs)*. Trondheim: St Olav Hospital.

Hadley, S. (1996) 'A rationale for the use of songs with children undergoing bone marrow transplantation.' *Australian Journal of Music Therapy 7*, 16–27.

Hallenbeck, J. (2002) 'Cross-cultural issues.' In A. Berger, R. Portenoy and D. Weissman (eds) *Principles and Practice of Palliative Care and Supportive Oncology*. New York: Lippincott, Williams and Wilkins.

Hilliard, R.E. (2001) 'The effects of music therapy-based bereavement groups on mood and behavior of grieving children: a pilot study.' *Journal of Music Therapy 38*, 4, 291–306.

Holland, J. (1996) 'Cancer's psychological challenges.' *Scientific American 275*, 3, 122–125.

Jones, A. and May, J. (1997) *Working in Human Service Organisations: A Critical Introduction*. Melbourne: Longman.

Kasher, A., Batori, G., Soroker, N., Graves, D. and Zaidel, E. (1999) 'Effects of right-and-left hemisphere damage on understanding conversational implicatures.' *Brain and Language 68*, 566–590.

Kennelly, J. (1999) 'Don't give up: providing music therapy to an adolescent boy in the bone marrow transplant unit.' In R.R. Pratt and D.E. Grocke (eds) *MusicMedicine 3: MusicMedicine and Music Therapy: Expanding Horizons*. Parkville, Victoria: Faculty of Music, University of Melbourne.

Klein, M. (1932) *The Psychoanalysis of Children*. London: Virago Press. (Original work published by Hogarth Press Ltd.)

Köster, W. (1997) *When Sunshine Gets Cold: Texte und Musik von krebskranken kindern und Jugendlichen*. KON 670–5 (CD).

Krout, R.E. (2000) 'Hospice and palliative music therapy: a continuum of creative caring.' In American Music Therapy Association (ed) *Effectiveness of Music Therapy Procedures: Documentation of Research and Clinical Practice*. Third edition. Silver Spring, MD: American Music Therapy Association Inc.

Krout, R.E. (2002) 'The use of therapist-composed songs to facilitate multi-modal grief processing and expression with bereaved children in group music therapy.' *Annual Journal of the New Zealand Society for Music Therapy*, 21–35.

Krout, R.E. (2003) 'Essential guitar skill development considerations for the contemporary music therapist.' *Music Therapy Today 4*, 2 (on-line) http://musictherapyworld.net

Krout, R.E. (2004) 'The use of directive lyric image and metaphor in therapist composed music and song with patients, families, staff and volunteers in palliative/hospice care.' Paper presented at the *Symposium on Music Therapy at the End of Life*, Beth Israel Medical Center, New York, March.

Krout, R.E. (in press[a]) 'Applications of music therapist-composed songs in creating participant connections and facilitating goals and rituals during one-time bereavement support groups and programs.' *Music Therapy Perspectives*.

Krout, R.E. (in press[b]) 'Therapist-composed music and song in end of life care.' In C. Dileo and J. Loewy (eds) *Music Therapy at the End of Life*. Cherry Hill, NJ: Jeffrey Publishers.

Laiho, S. (2004) 'The psychological functions of music in adolescence.' *Nordic Journal of Music Therapy 13*, 1, 47–63.

Lambert, M.J. and Ogles, B.M. (2004) 'The efficacy and effectiveness of psychotherapy.' In M.J. Lambert (ed) *Bergin and Garfield's Handbook of Psychotherapy and Behavior Change*. Fifth edition. New York: John Wiley and Sons Inc.

Lane, D. (1988) 'Music therapy and oncology patients: the challenge and the response.' Paper presented at the *Symposium on Music Therapy with the Terminally Ill: The Next Step Forward*, New York.

Lane, D. (1992) 'Music therapy: a gift beyond measure.' *Oncology Nursing Forum 19*, 6, 863–867.

Lang, P.H. (1941) *Music in Western Civilization*. New York: Norton and Co.

Laplanche, J. and Pontalis, J.B. (1973) *The Language of Psychoanalysis*. London: Karnac Books.

Lavigne, A. (29 May–4 June 2004) Interview in *Hot Stars* magazine pp.44–47.

Ledger, A. (2001) 'Song parody for adolescents with cancer.' *The Australian Journal of Music Therapy 12*, 21–27.

Lee, K. and Baker, F. (1997) 'Towards integrating a holistic rehabilitation system: the implications for music therapy.' *Australian Journal of Music Therapy 8*, 30–37.

Leigh, S. and Clark, E. (2002) 'Psychosocial aspects of cancer survivorship.' In A. Berger, R. Portenoy and D. Weissman (eds) *Principles of Practice of Palliative Care and Supportive Oncology*. New York: Lippincott, Williams and Wilkins.

Lindberg, K.A. (1995) 'Songs of healing: songwriting with an abused adolescent.' *Music Therapy 13*, 1, 93–108.

Living Soul (2004) Triple CD produced by Emma O'Brien and Nigel Derricks, Melbourne. Distributed by MGM. www.mh.org.au/livingsoul

Lord, C., Rutter, M., Goode, S., Heemsberger, J., Jordan, H., Mawhood, L. and Schopler, E. (1989) 'Autistic diagnostic observation schedule: a standardised observation of communicative and social behaviour.' *Journal of Autism and Developmental Disorders 19*, 2, 185–212.

Maciszewski, A. (2000) 'About the music of India.' www.io.com/~peterc/talla.html

Magill, L. (2005) 'Music therapy and spirituality at the end-of-life.' In C. Dileo and J. Loewy (eds) *Music Therapy at the End of Life*. Cherry Hill, NJ: Jeffrey Books.

Magill, L. and Luzzatto, P. (2002) 'Music therapy and art therapy.' In A. Berger, R. Portenoy and D. Weissman (eds) *Principles and Practice of Palliative Care and Supportive Oncology*. New York: Lippincott, Williams and Wilkins.

Magill-Levreault, L. (1993) 'Music therapy in pain and symptom management.' *Journal of Palliative Care 9*, 4, 42–48.

Mandel, S.E. (1991) 'Music therapy in the hospice: musicalive.' *Palliative Medicine 5*, 155–160.

McFerran, K. (2003) 'Active methods for working with adolescents: a comparison of songwriting and improvisation.' Unpublished paper presented at the *Fourth Nordic Music Therapy Conference*, Bergen.

McFerran, K. (in press) 'Using songs with groups of teenagers: how does it work?' *Social Works With Groups 27*, 2.

McFerran-Skewes, K. and Grocke, D.E. (2000) 'What do grieving young people and music therapy have in common? Exploring the match between creativity and younger adolescents.' *European Journal of Palliative Care 7*, 6, 227–230.

Mechanic, D. (1999) 'Mental health and mental illness: definitions and perspectives.' In A. Horwitz and T.L. Scheid (eds) *A Handbook for the Study of Mental Health: Social Contexts, Theories, and Systems*. Cambridge: Cambridge University Press.

Melamed, B. (1992) 'Family factors predicting children's reactions to anesthesia induction.' In A.M. La Greca (ed) *Stress and Coping in Child Health*. New York: The Guilford Press.

Montello, L. (2003) 'Protect this child: psychodynamic music therapy with a gifted musician.' In S. Hadley (ed) *Psychodynamic Music Therapy: Case Studies*. Gilsum, NH: Barcelona Publishers.

Moore, R. (2003) *Ethnomusicology Workshop*, Temple University.

Mullen, P.E., Martin, J.L., Anderson, J.C., Romons, S.E. and Herbison, G.P. (1996) 'The long-term impact of the physical, emotional and sexual abuse of children: a community study.' *Child Abuse and Neglect 20*, 1, 7–21.

Nolan, P. (1992) 'Music therapy with bone marrow transplant patients: reaching beyond the symptoms.' In R. Spintge and R. Droh (eds) *MusicMedicine*. St Louis: MMB Music.

Nolan, P. (1998) 'Countertransference in clinical songwriting.' In K. Bruscia (ed) *The Dynamics of Music Psychotherapy*. Gilsum, NH: Barcelona Publishers.

Nordenfelt, L. (1987) *On the Nature of Health: An Action-Theoretic Approach*. Dodrecht: D. Reidel Publishing Company.

Nordoff, P. and Robbins, C. (1983) *Music Therapy in Special Education*. Second edition. St Louis: MMB Music.

O'Brien, E. (1999a) 'Cancer patients' evaluation of a music therapy program in a public adult hospital.' In R.R. Pratt and D.E. Grocke (eds) *MusicMedicine 3: MusicMedicine and Music Therapy: Expanding Horizons*. Parkville, Victoria: Faculty of Music, University of Melbourne.

O'Brien, E.K. (1999b) 'The experience of song writing and song sharing in cancer care.' Paper presented at the *Ninth World Congress of Music Therapy*, Washington, USA.

O'Brien, E.K. (2003) 'The nature of the interactions between patient and therapist when writing a song on a bone marrow transplant ward.' Unpublished masters thesis, The University of Melbourne.

O'Brien, E. (2004) 'The language of guided song writing with a bone marrow transplant patient.' *Voices 4*, 1, http://www.voices.no/mainissues/mi40004000139p.html

O'Brien, W. (1991) 'Making parent education relevant to vulnerable parents.' *Children Australia 16*, 2, 19–26.

O'Callaghan, C. (1990) 'Music therapy skills used in song-writing within a palliative care setting.' *The Australian Journal of Music Therapy 1*, 15–22.

O'Callaghan, C. (1996) 'Lyrical themes in songs written by palliative care patients.' *Journal of Music Therapy 33*, 2, 74–92.

O'Callaghan, C. (1997) 'Therapeutic opportunities associated with the music when using song writing in palliative care.' *Music Therapy Perspectives 15*, 1, 32–38.

O'Callaghan, C. (2001) 'Music therapy's relevance in a cancer hospital researched through a constructivist's lens.' Unpublished PhD thesis, The University of Melbourne.

O'Connor, A., Wicker, C. and Germino, B. (1990) 'Understanding the cancer patient's search for meaning.' *Cancer Nursing 13*, 3, 167–175.

Oldfield, A. (1993) 'Music therapy with families.' In M. Heal and T. Wigram (eds) *Music Therapy in Health and Education*. London: Jessica Kingsley Publishers.

Oldfield, A. (2000) 'Music therapy as a contribution to the diagnosis made by the staff team in child and family psychiatry: an initial description of a methodology that is still emerging through clinical practice.' In T. Wigram (ed) *Assessment and Evaluation in the Arts Therapies*. St Albans, UK: Harper House Publications.

Oldfield, A. (2004) 'Music therapy with children on the autistic spectrum: approaches derived from clinical practice and research.' Unpublished PhD thesis, Anglia Polytechnic University, Cambridge, Great Britain.

Olney, M.F. and Kim, A. (2001) 'Beyond adjustment: integration of cognitive disability into identity.' *Disability and Society 16*, 4, 563–583.

Palmer, N. (1991) 'Making parent education relevant to vulnerable parents.' *Children Australia 16*, 2, 19–26.

Pavlicevic, M. and Ansdell, G. (2004) 'The ripple effect.' In M. Pavlicevic and G. Ansdell (eds) *Community Music Therapy*. London: Jessica Kingsley Publishers.

Plessen, C. von (1995) 'Krankheitserfahrungen von krebskranken Kindern und ihren Familien.' Inagural-Dissertation. Universität Witten/Herdecke.

Post-White, J., Ceronsky, C., Kreitzer, M.J., Nickelson, K., Drew, D., Mackey, K.W., Koopmeiners, L. and Gutknecht, S. (1996) 'Hope, spirituality, sense of coherence, and quality of life in patients with cancer.' *Oncology Nurses Forum 23*, 10, 1571–1579.

Priestley, M. (1998) *Essays on Analytical Music Therapy*. Phoenixville: Barcelona Publishers.

Primadei, A. (2004) 'The use of the guitar in clinical improvisation.' *Music Therapy Today* (online) 5, 4 (August). Available at http://musictherapyworld.net

Radocy, R.E. and Boyle, J.D. (2003) *Psychological Foundations of Musical Behavior*. Fourth edition. Springfield, IL: Charles C. Thomas.

Ricciarelli, A. (2003) 'The guitar in palliative music therapy for cancer patients.' *Music Therapy Today* (online) 4, 2. Available at http://musictherapyworld.net

Robarts, J. (2003) 'The healing function of improvised songs in music therapy with a child survivor of early trauma and sexual abuse.' In S. Hadley (ed) *Psychodynamic Music Therapy: Case Studies*. Gilsum, NH: Barcelona Publishers.

Robb, S. (1996) 'Techniques in song writing: restoring emotional and physical wellbeing in adolescents who have been traumatically injured.' *Music Therapy Perspectives 14*, 30–37.

Robb, S.L. and Ebberts, A.G. (2003a) 'Song writing and digital video production interventions for pediatric patients undergoing bone marrow transplantation, Part I: An analysis of depression and anxiety levels according to phase of treatment.' *Journal of Pediatric Oncology Nursing 20*, 1, 2–15.

Robb, S.L. and Ebberts, A.G. (2003b) 'Song writing and digital video production interventions for pediatric patients undergoing bone marrow transplantation, Part II: An analysis of patient-generated songs and patient perceptions regarding intervention efficacy.' *Journal of Pediatric Oncology Nursing 20*, 1, 16–25.

Robertson-Gilliam, K. (1995) 'The role of music therapy in meeting the spiritual needs of the dying person.' In C.A. Lee (ed) *Lonely Waters*. Oxford: Sobell Publications.

Rogers, P. (2003) 'Working with Jenny: stories of gender, power and abuse.' In S. Hadley (ed) *Psychodynamic Music Therapy: Case Studies*. Gilsum, NH: Barcelona Publishers.

Rolvsjord, R. (2001) 'Sophie learns to play her songs of tears.' *Nordic Journal of Music Therapy 10*, 1, 77–86.

Rolvsjord, R. (2003) 'Resource-oriented music therapy in psychiatry – a Norwegian way?' Paper presented at the *Fourth Nordic Music Therapy Conference*, Bergen.

Rolvsjord, R. (2004) Empowerment as metaphor for therapy. Paper presented at the *Seventh European Music Therapy Conference*, Jyväskylä.

Romanowski, B. (2003) 'Men and guitars: personal experience with the guitar in music therapy.' *Music Therapy Today* (online) 4, 2 (April). Available at http://musictherapyworld.net

Rooksby, R. (2000) *How to Write Songs on Guitar*. San Francisco: Backbeat Books.

Round, C. (2001) 'An exploration of the role and function of music therapy in a multidisciplinary service for adolescents.' Unpublished MA thesis, Anglia Polytechnic University.

Ruud, E. (1998) *Music Therapy: Improvisation, Communication and Culture*. Pheonixville: Barcelona Publishers.

Sachs, C. (1969) *A Short History of World Music*. London: Dobson Books.

Sadie, S. (1980) *The New Groves Dictionary of Music and Musicians*, Vol. 17. London: Macmillan Publishers.

Saleebey, D. (2002) *Strengths Perspective in Social Work Practice*. Boston: Allyn and Bacon.

Salmon, D. (1993) 'Music and emotion in palliative care.' *Journal of Palliative Care 9*, 4, 48–52.

Schmidt, J.A. (1983) 'Songwriting as a therapeutic procedure.' *Music Therapy Perspectives 1*, 2, 4–7.

Seager, K.M. and Spencer, S.C. (1996) 'Meeting the bereavement needs of kids in patient/families: not just kidding around.' *Hospice Journal 11*, 4, 41–66.

Sheridan, J. and McFerran, K. (2004) 'Exploring the value of opportunities for choice and control in music therapy within a paediatric hospice setting.' *The Australian Journal of Music Therapy 15*, 18–32.

Silber, F. and Hes, J.P. (1995) 'The use of songwriting with patients diagnosed with Alzheimer's disease.' *Music Therapy Perspectives 13*, 1, 31–34.

Simpson, G., Simons, M. and McFadyen, M. (2002) 'The challenges of a hidden disability: social work practice in the field of traumatic brain injury.' *Australian Social Work 55*, 1, 24–37.

Skewes, K. and Grocke, D.E. (2000) 'What does group music therapy offer to bereaved young people? A rounded approach to the grieving adolescent.' *Grief Matters: The Australian Journal of Loss and Grief 3*, 3, 54–61.

Slivka, H. and Magill, L. (1986) 'The conjoint use of social work and music therapy with children of cancer patients.' *Music Therapy 6A*, 1, 30–40.

Smith, G.H. (1991) 'The song-writing process: a woman's struggle against depression and suicide.' In K. Bruscia (ed) *Case Studies in Music Therapy*. Phoenixville: Barcelona Publishers.

Smyth, M. (2002) 'The role of creativity in healing and recovering one's power after victimisation.' In J. Sutton (ed) *Music, Music Therapy and Trauma: International Perspectives*. London: Jessica Kingsley Publishers.

Stainer, J. and Barrett, W.A. (1875) *Dictionary of Musical Terms*. London: Novello.

Standley, J. (1986) 'Music research in medical/dental treatment: meta-analysis and clinical applications.' *Journal of Music Therapy 23*, 56–122.

Stige, B. (2002) *Culture-Centred Music Therapy*. Gilsum, NH: Barcelona Publishers.

Storr, A. (1992) *Music and the Mind*. London: HarperCollins.

Tallman, K. and Bohart, A.C. (1999) 'The client as a common factor: clients as self-healers.' In M.A. Hubble, B.L. Duncan and S.D. Miller (eds) *The Heart and Soul of Change: What Works in Psychotherapy*. Washington: American Psychological Association.

Teahan, M. (2000) 'Grief interventions.' In M. Teahan and T. Dalton (eds) *Helping Children and Adolescents Cope with Grief and Bereavement*. Symposium conducted at the Alumni Conference of the Barry University School of Social Work, Miami, FL.

Todres, R. and Wojtiuk, R. (1979) 'The cancer patient's view of chemotherapy.' *Cancer Nursing 8*, 283–573.

Turry, A. (1999) 'A song of life: improvised songs with children with cancer and serious blood disorders.' In T. Wigram and J. De Backer (eds) *Clinical Applications of Music Therapy in Developmental Disability, Paediatrics, and Neurology*. London: Jessica Kingsley Publishers.

Vermeulen, P. (2001) *Autistic Thinking – This is the Title*. London: Jessica Kingsley Publishers.

Vetesse, J. (1976) 'Problems of the patient confronting the diagnosis of cancer.' In J.W. Cullen, B.H. Fox and R.N. Isom (eds) *Cancer: The Behavioural Dimensions*. New York: Raven Press.

Wampold, B.E. (2001) *The Great Psychotherapy Debate: Models, Methods, and Findings*. London: Lawrence Erlbaum Associates.

Watts, S. (2003) *Ethomusicology Workshop*, Temple University.

Weber, S., Nuessler, V. and Wilmanns, W. (1997) 'A pilot study on the influence of receptive music listening on cancer patients during chemotherapy.' *International Journal of Arts Medicine 5*, 27–35.

Wechsler, D. (1992) *Wechsler Intelligence Scale for Children*. Third edition. London: The Psychological Corporation.

Wigram, T. (2004) *Improvisation: Methods and Techniques for Music Therapy Clinicians, Educators and Students*. London: Jessica Kingsley Publishers.

Wigram, T., Pedersen, I.N. and Bonde, L.O. (2002) *A Comprehensive Guide to Music Therapy Theory, Clinical Practice, Research and Training*. London: Jessica Kingsley Publishers.

Wright, B.A. (1960) *Physical Disability: A Psychological Approach*. New York and Evanston: Harper and Row.

Yalom, I.D. (1995) *The Theory and Practice of Group Psychotherapy*. Fourth edition. New York: Basic Books.

Contributors

Trygve Aasgaard is lecturer in music therapy at the Norwegian Academy of Music and Associate Professor at Oslo University College, where he teaches various subjects related to music, health and palliative care. His PhD dissertation (Aalborg University, Denmark) was a longitudinal study of the 'life histories' of songs made and performed by seriously ill children alone or together with the music therapist and others. In the mid-1990s he established and developed music therapy services at Hospice Lovisenberg and at the paediatric departments of the National Hospital (Rikshospitalet) and Ulleval University Hospital, Oslo. He has written various papers and chapters relating to community music therapy, songwriting, qualitative case study research and health issues, especially related to children and adults with life threatening diseases. His many-sided compositional expereinces include film music and works for string orchestra and big band.

Felicity Baker is head of the music therapy training programme at the University of Queensland, Brisbane, Australia. She graduated from her undergraduate music therapy training from Melbourne University in 1992 and then with a master's research degree in 1999. She defended her PhD thesis in May 2004 at Aalborg University, Denmark. In 1993 Felicity developed the first post in music therapy in the area of brain injury rehabilitation in Australia and she has researched and published extensively in this area. She has developed a particular interest in how music therapy can facilitate improvements in communication for this population. Felicity is currently editorial board member of the *Nordic Journal of Music Therapy* and reviewer for the *Australian Journal of Music Therapy*. She has been active within the Australian Music Therapy Association, including serving terms as Vice President, President and Past President.

Emma Davies trained as a music therapist at Anglia Polytechnic University, Cambridge, in 2000. Since then she has worked at the Croft Unit for Child and Family Psychiatry and at the Child Development Centre, Addenbrooke's Hospital, Cambridge. She has also set up a variety of music therapy projects within Early Years settings and in the community, working for the Cambridgeshire Instrumental Music Agency and for SureStart. She has a particular interest in working with children and their families and was a research assistant on a PhD project investigating music therapy for children on the autistic spectrum.

Toni Day is a registered music therapist who has had extensive clinical experience working with a wide range of populations. She is currently the Co-ordinator of Clinical Training at the University of Queensland, where she is responsible for all aspects of the clinical training component of the programme, from establishing new training opportunities for music therapy students through to supervising students and the training of music therapy clinical educators. She began her career working within aged care, and since then has gained experience working within the disability fields with children and adults with varying degrees of neurological and physical impairments. Toni has more recently specialized in working in private practice with children with autistic spectrum disorder and with women and children who have experienced childhood trauma and/or domestic violence. She is currently studying her master's research degree, investigating the role of therapeutic song writing for women who have experienced childhood abuse, and has recently published on her work with refugee young people.

Philippa Derrington, BA(Hons), DipMth, studied and taught modern languages both in the UK and abroad before training as a music therapist at Anglia Polytechnic University. After qualifying in 2001, she worked with children with special needs and emotional and behavioural difficulties in schools across Cambridgeshire and Bedfordshire and as part of the outreach music therapy team at the children's hospice in Cambridge. She has pioneered and established a music therapy provision at a mainstream secondary school. She presented this work at the European Congress of Music Therapy in 2004 and is currently doing an MA which examines the role of music therapy in this setting.

Cheryl Dileo, PhD, MT-BC, is Professor of Music Therapy at Temple University, Philadelphia. She currently coordinates the Master's Program in Music Therapy, the music therapy clinical programmes at Temple University Hospital and is a music therapist at Compassionate Care Hospice. In addition, she is the Director of the new, interdisciplinary Arts and Quality of Life Research Center. She has served in a variety of leadership positions for the World Federation of Music Therapy, including President, Past-President and Chair of the Commission on Ethics, and currently she holds the position of Business Manager. She developed the WFMT Guidelines for Ethics. She has also held a variety of leadership positions in the National Association for Music Therapy, including President, Vice President and Council Coordinator. She played a leading role in the development of the NAMT Code of Ethics, and currently is Co-Chair of AMTA's Ethics Board. She has given more than 200 lectures and workshops in this country and abroad, having conducted lecture tours in 17 countries on 5 continents. She was named the McAndless Distinguished Scholar and Professor in the Humanities for the 2002–3 academic year at Eastern Michigan University. She has served on the Editorial Board of the *Journal of Music Therapy* and *Music Therapy: The Journal of the American Association for Music Therapy*. She is currently a consulting editor for the *International Journal of Arts in Psychotherapy*. She serves as a grant consultant for the National Institute of Health, the National Center for Complementary and Alternative Medicine, and the National Cancer Institute. She is the author/editor of 12 books and 80 articles and book chapters.

Christine Franke is a Psychoanalytic Psychotherapist working with adults in private practice in Bedfordshire. She is doing a PhD at the Centre for Psychoanalytic Studies, Essex University. Her research has involved making observations of children on the autistic spectrum, in various settings in the Croft Unit, to see how they express, process and regulate emotions.

Jeanette Kennelly is Senior Music Therapist at the Royal Children's Hospital, Brisbane, Australia, where she works in the rehabilitation unit. Her clinical practice and research in paediatrics has been widely published nationally and internationally throughout well known music therapy, nursing and other health-related refereed journals. The main focus of her publications has been neurorehabilitation, in particular the interface of music therapy and speech pathology in paediatric rehabilitation.

Robert E. Krout, Ed.D, MT-BC, RMTh, is Head of Music Therapy at Southern Methodist University in Dallas, Texas. He received a Bachelor of Music in Music Education from Ithaca College, and a Master of Arts in Music Therapy, Master of Education in Special Education, and Doctor of Education in Music Education and Therapy from Columbia University-Teacher's College. He has worked as a music therapist since 1980 in a variety of settings, including public schools, state institutions, hospitals, summer camps, hospices and bereavement centres. He has taught at several universities, including from 1982 to 1997 at SUNY New Paltz. At the Hospice of Palm Beach County, Florida, he was Music Therapy Manager and Internship Director. From July 2002 to July 2004, he taught at Massey University in New Zealand – that country's first dedicated university music therapy programme. Recent, current and in press journal publications include those in the *American Journal of Hospice & Palliative Care, American Journal of Recreation Therapy, The Arts in Psychotherapy, Australian Journal of Music Therapy, Music Therapy Perspectives* and *New Zealand Journal of Music Therapy*. Robert's current clinical work is with Camp Sol in Dallas, a non-profit organization providing interdisciplinary grief services for bereaved families who still have children 18 and younger at home.

Lucanne Magill, DA(ABD), MT-BC, is Manager of the Music Therapy Program, Integrative Medicine Service, Memorial Sloan-Kettering Cancer Center, New York, where she provides music therapy to patients, families and staff, supervises music therapy interns and coordinates hospital-wide music therapy programmes. She has been working closely with cancer patients and families since 1973 and developed Memorial Sloan-Kettering's music therapy programme. She has conducted research, lectured internationally and has published numerous articles and chapters on topics relating to music therapy and cancer. She is a workshop leader for Cancer Care in New York City and is currently a Doctoral candidate at New York University. She is a per diem music therapist for Cabrini Hospice in New York City where she is also conducting research on music therapy and spirituality.

Emma O'Brien, BMus, RMT, MMus, established the position of music therapist at the Royal Melbourne Hospital in June 1997, practising in oncology, palliative care, bone marrow transplant and early psychosis. More recently she has begun a group music programme in the eating disorders unit (http://www.mh.org.au/sitesandservices/MusicTherapy/default.htm). Emma has presented her clinical practice and research at many national and international conferences, and has had her work published in peer reviewed texts. She is a casual lecturer at the University of Melbourne in voice and songwriting in music therapy methods. Emma completed her master's thesis in songwriting with bone marrow transplant patients in 2003. She regularly gives seminars on music therapy to community groups. Emma recorded, with professional musicians, and produced, with Nigel Derricks, the groundbreaking triple CD project *Living Soul* – songs written in music therapy practice with people whose lives are touched by cancer (www.mh.org.au/livingsoul). It is available commercially.

Amelia Oldfield has worked as a music therapist in Cambridge for the past 24 years. She currently works at the Croft Unit for Child and Family Psychiatry and at the Child Development Centre, Addenbrooke's. She was the joint initiator of the MA Music Therapy Training at Anglia Polytechnic University, where she is a part-time lecturer. She has researched music therapy for adults with severe learning difficulties (MPhil), music therapy for parents and young children, and music therapy for children on the autistic spectrum (PhD). She writes and lectures extensively on many aspects of music therapy and has produced five music therapy training videos.

Randi Rolvsjord is assistant professor at the music therapy programme in Sandane, Sogn og Fjordane University College, Norway. She also works as a music therapist at a psychiatric centre in Nordfjordeid. She is a PhD student at Aalborg University, doing her doctoral research on 'Resource-oriented music therapy in psychiatry'.

Jeanette Tamplin, BMus(Hons), RMT, NMT, is Senior Music Therapist at the Royal Talbot Rehabilitation Centre, Austin Health, and works as a consultant music therapist at other rehabilitation hospitals in Melbourne. She has over seven years' experience working in neurorehabilitation and has published on her work in this area. Jeanette is currently completing a master's by research degree in Music Therapy at the University of Melbourne in the area of acquired communication disorders. She has served for four years in various capacities on the National Council of AMTA, including terms as National Secretary and National Treasurer.

Tony Wigram is Professor of Music Therapy and Head of PhD Studies in Music Therapy at the Institute for Music and Music Therapy, Department of Humanities, University of Aalborg, Denmark. He is Head Music Therapist at the Harper House Children's Service, Hertfordshire, England, Research Advisor to Hertfordshire Partnership NHS Trust, and a Research Fellow in the Faculty of Music, Melbourne University. He was Churchill Fellow of 1985, and in 2004 was awarded the first European Music Therapy Confederation Award for significant contributions to the development of music therapy in Europe. He is a Former President of the European Music Therapy Confederation and of the World Federation of Music Therapy. He studied music therapy under Juliette Alvin, psychology at Royal Holloway, and wrote his doctoral thesis in Psychology at St George's Medical School, London University. He has supervised more than 12 doctoral studies in music therapy, and is Academic Coordinator at the International Graduate School of Doctoral Research at Aalborg University, Denmark. He is a Visiting Professor in Music Therapy at Anglia Polytechnic University, Cambridge, ISFOM, Naples, Italy, and the Escuela de Musicoterapia, Vitoria-Gasteiz, Spain, as well as regularly teaching in Belgium, Australia and the US. He has written or edited 13 books on music therapy and authored more than 100 articles in peer reviewed journals and chapters in books. His research interests include the physiological effect of sound and music, assessment and diagnosis of pervasive developmental disorders, Rett syndrome, methods of advanced level improvisation, and research training in music therapy.

Subject Index

12-bar blues 15, 235

accompaniment
    adding additional 221–2
    art of 158, 164–5
    choice of instrument 216
    methods of guiding 199–202
    setting 193, 203–4, 261
acoustic guitar 217
acting out 73, 258
adjustment, traumatic brain injury 116–18
    inhibitors 119–21
adolescents
    songwriting as therapy for 14–15
    see also teenagers
adult oncology patients 180–205
    diagnosis of cancer 181
    songwriting with 15, 181–2
        GOLM method see Guiding Original
            Lyrics and Music
    see also multicultural oncology patients
adult psychiatric patients
    musical interaction 97–8
    songwriting with 15, 98–9
        case examples 103–14
        co-creations of lyrics 101
        co-creations of songs from clients'
            poems 101–3
        method and techniques 100
        therapeutic functions 114–15
adult survivors, child abuse
    impact of abuse 82–3
    songwriting
        brainstorming on themes 87
        case example 91–5
        lyric creation 87–8
        methodological orientation 84
        music creation 88–9
        programmes 85–6
        rationale for using 83–4
        rehearsing and recording 89–91
        steps involved in 86–7
African-American musical forms 235–7
Allan 29, 38
Alvin model, improvisation 69–70
Ana 241–4
aphasia 119
arousal, heightened 27
audio-recordings 161
Autism Diagnostic Interview 26

Autism Diagnostic Observation Schedule 26
autistic children, lack of internal world 43

Be all right 208–9, 210–22
Be with me now 111–14
bereaved teenagers, songwriting with 207–23
    addressing clinical need 210–12
    deciding who is to write the song and why
        212–13
    determining which will come first, lyrics
        or music 213
    roughing out the lyrics for content
        214–15
    choosing style and feel of the song
        216–17
    lyric rhythm and rhyme 217–18
    chord progression 218–20
    adding the melody over the chords 220–1
    verse-chorus song form 221
    additional accompaniment and stylistic
        features 221
black humour, in songs 169
blues song form 15, 235–7
bone marrow transplantation 155–6
boredom 36
Boy Band style, case example 146–50
brainstorming
    ideas and themes 50, 56, 87, 139, 185–7,
        203, 258
    towards a song structure 187
bridges, in songs 188, 221

C major introduction 30–1
call and response techniques 237
cancer
    diagnosis and treatment of 181
    patients see adult oncology patients; child
        oncology patients
chants, East Indian 237–44
chase sound effects 31
chemotherapy 155
child abuse see adult survivors; sexual abuse
child oncology patients
    music therapy
        limitations and challenges 155–6
        technical equipment 156
    songwriting
        health perspective on 154–5
        working methods and principles
            157–79
child psychiatric patients
    music therapy diagnostic assessments
        26–8

276

Author Index